D1188623

CONTROVERSIES IN THE DETERMINATION OF DEATH

CONTROVERSIES IN THE DETERMINATION OF DEATH

A White Paper of
the President's Council on Bioethics

Washington, DC
December 2008

www.bioethics.gov

CONTENTS

⧉⧉

LETTER OF TRANSMITTAL TO THE PRESIDENT OF THE UNITED STATES

The President's Council on Bioethics
1425 New York Avenue, NW, Suite C100
Washington, DC 20005
December 2008

The President
The White House
Washington, DC

Dear Mr. President:

I am pleased to present to you a white paper by the President's Council on Bioethics entitled *Controversies in the Determination of Death*. It is the report of an inquiry that was occasioned by another forthcoming Council report on ethical questions in organ transplantation. The two reports are linked ethically: most of the organs procured for transplantation in this country come from deceased donors who have been declared dead in accord with the neurological standard.

This white paper by the Council is primarily concerned with a careful analysis of the ethical questions raised by the neurological standard, i.e., the clinical determination of "whole brain death." This standard was defended in 1981 by the President's Commission for the Study of Ethical Problems in Medicine and Biomedical and Behavioral Research. In that report, the Commission also proposed a model statute to foster uniformity in law and medical practice nationwide. Since then, the neurological standard has been accepted as one of two valid standards for determining death and has been adopted in many countries throughout the world. (The other accepted standard is the older, traditional cardiopulmonary standard.)

In recent years, however, controversy has arisen about the clinical and ethical validity of the neurological standard. Some think it too restrictive to meet the need for transplantable organs; others fear that "whole brain death" may not be the equivalent of the death of the human being; still others believe that, in the face of any uncertainty, it is ethically prudent to re-examine the concept and the evidence critically.

In this white paper, the Council has given careful consideration to contending positions in this controversy. After reviewing the relevant literature and the testimony of many experts, followed by intensive discussion between and among its members, the Council has concluded that the neurological standard remains valid. Some Council members, however, believe that a better philosophical rationale than the one proposed by the President's Commission of 1981 should be adopted. A few Council members argue that there is sufficient uncertainty about the neurological standard to warrant an alternative approach to the care of the "brain dead" human being and the question of organ procurement.

The Council presents this study in the spirit of your original Executive Order to "...facilitate a greater understanding of bioethical issues." By re-examining the neurological standard and placing it within its clinical, historical, and ethical context and by critically analyzing arguments for and against its validity, the Council believes it has fulfilled this mandate. The Council also hopes that this white paper will help the public and its policymakers to reflect on a matter of profound human significance in such a way that the dignity of the human person will be preserved. Only in this way can the benefits of modern technology be realized within ethical constraints.

Sincerely,

Edmund D. Pellegrino, M.D.
Chairman

MEMBERS OF
THE PRESIDENT'S COUNCIL ON BIOETHICS

EDMUND D. PELLEGRINO, M.D., CHAIRMAN
Professor Emeritus of Medicine and Medical Ethics, and Adjunct Professor of Philosophy, Georgetown University

FLOYD E. BLOOM, M.D.
Professor Emeritus in the Molecular and Integrative Neuroscience Department at The Scripps Research Institute

BENJAMIN S. CARSON, SR., M.D.
The Benjamin S. Carson, Sr., M.D., and Dr. Evelyn Spiro, R.N., Professor of Pediatric Neurosurgery, Director of Pediatric Neurosurgery, and Professor of Neurosurgery, Oncology, Plastic Surgery, and Pediatrics, Johns Hopkins Medical Institutions

REBECCA S. DRESSER, J.D., M.S.
Daniel Noyes Kirby Professor of Law and Professor of Ethics in Medicine, Washington University, St. Louis

NICHOLAS N. EBERSTADT, PH.D.
Henry Wendt Chair in Political Economy, American Enterprise Institute

JEAN B. ELSHTAIN, PH.D.
Laura Spelman Rockefeller Professor of Social and Political Ethics, University of Chicago, and Thomas and Dorothy Leavey Chair in the Foundation of American Freedom, Georgetown University

DANIEL W. FOSTER, M.D.
John Denis McGarry, Ph.D., Distinguished Chair in Diabetes and Metabolic Research, University of Texas Southwestern Medical Center, Dallas, TX

MICHAEL S. GAZZANIGA, PH.D.
Director of Sage Center for the Study of Mind, University of California, Santa Barbara

ROBERT P. GEORGE, J.D., D.PHIL.
McCormick Professor of Jurisprudence and Director of the James Madison Program in American Ideals and Institutions, Princeton University

ALFONSO GÓMEZ-LOBO, DR. PHIL.
Ryan Family Professor of Metaphysics and Moral Philosophy, Georgetown University

WILLIAM B. HURLBUT, M.D.
Consulting Professor, Neurology and Neurological Sciences, Stanford Medical Center, Stanford University

DONALD W. LANDRY, M.D., PH.D.
Professor of Medicine, Director of the Division of Experimental Therapeutics, and Chair, Department of Medicine, Columbia University

PETER A. LAWLER, PH.D.
Dana Professor and Chair of the Department of Government and International Studies, Berry College

PAUL R. MCHUGH, M.D.
University Distinguished Service Professor of Psychiatry, The Johns Hopkins University School of Medicine

GILBERT C. MEILAENDER, PH.D.
Richard and Phyllis Duesenberg Professor of Christian Ethics, Valparaiso University

JANET D. ROWLEY, M.D.
Blum-Riese Distinguished Service Professor of Medicine, of Molecular Genetics and Cell Biology, and of Human Genetics, Pritzker School of Medicine, University of Chicago

DIANA J. SCHAUB, PH.D.
Professor of Political Science, Loyola College

CARL E. SCHNEIDER, J.D.
Chauncey Stillman Professor of Ethics, Morality, and the Practice of Law, and Professor of Internal Medicine, University of Michigan

COUNCIL STAFF

F. Daniel Davis, Ph.D.
Executive Director

Judith E. Crawford
Administrative Director

Samuel J. Crowe, Ph.D.
Deputy Director

Diane M. Gianelli
Director of Communications

Ginger Gruters
Research Assistant

Emily L. Jones
Executive Administrator

Audrea V. Medina
Information Technology
Specialist

Thomas W. Merrill, Ph.D.
Senior Research Analyst

David G. Miller, Ph.D.
Senior Research Analyst

Marti Patchell
Special Assistant to the
Chairman

Joseph A. Raho
Research Assistant

Alan Rubenstein
Senior Consultant

Adam Schulman, Ph.D.
Senior Research Consultant

CONTROVERSIES IN THE DETERMINATION OF DEATH

PREFACE

The question of how—by what standard—an individual should be declared dead is once more a matter of controversy. With this report, the President's Council on Bioethics takes up this controversy and seeks to illuminate the issues at the center of the renewed debate about the inherently perplexing problems of determining human death in an age of life-sustaining technologies. In the following pages, the President's Council examines the main lines of criticism and defense of the neurological standard, and also explores the ethical concerns engendered by the use of the traditional cardiopulmonary standard in the organ procurement practice known as "controlled donation after cardiac death." In so doing, the President's Council on Bioethics aims to apprise the American public of the contemporary state of the debate and to guide the public's reflections on matters that touch on some of society's deepest human questions.

CHAPTER ONE

INTRODUCTION

In the late twentieth century, as a response to certain advances in critical care medicine, a new standard for determining death became accepted in both the medical and legal communities in the United States and many other parts of the world. Until then, the prevailing standard was the traditional cardiopulmonary standard: the irreversible loss of heart and lung functions signals the death of a human being. The new standard, which took its place alongside the traditional one, is based on the irreversible loss of all brain-dependent functions. In most human deaths, the loss of these neurological functions is accompanied by the traditional, familiar markers of death: the patient stops breathing, his or her heart stops beating, and the body starts to decay. In relatively rare cases, however, the irreversible loss of brain-dependent functions occurs while the body, with technological assistance, continues to circulate blood and to show other signs of life. In such cases, there is controversy and confusion about whether death has actually occurred.

There is controversy as well about the use of the traditional cardiopulmonary standard in the organ procurement practice known as "controlled donation after cardiac death" (controlled DCD). Here, too, there is debate about whether, at the time that organs are taken, the donor is truly dead. But, with controlled DCD, there is also a more acute danger that the quality of end-of-life care for the patient-donor will be compromised.

The controversies surrounding both the neurological standard and controlled DCD are the subject of this report, although the report's primary focus is the resurgent debate about the ethical validity of the neurological standard. Forty years after its inception, long-standing doubts about the standard's biological basis, fueled by ·more recent clinical observations about patients diagnosed as "brain dead," have reignited the debate about the standard's validity.

I. The History of the Neurological Standard for Determining Death

It was a key advance in medical technology—the mechanical ventilator—that originally gave rise to the confusions and controversies about when death occurs in a critical care setting. A review of the history of the neurological standard for death will help to explain why.

A. The Ventilator and the Problem of Determining Death

The mechanical ventilator externally supports the patient's *breathing* when injury or infirmity prevents the body from doing this vital work on its own. The injuries and diseases that might lead to a need for such support are many and varied. The incapacity to breathe on one's own is a common endpoint of different ailments and, of course, a terminal one unless help can be provided quickly. Although it does not treat the underlying disease, the ventilator may stave off death, often for months or even years.

Soon after the ventilator began to be used in hospitals all over the world, a set of ethical and philosophical complexities became evident. One involved the question of whether maintaining a patient on a ventilator is always in the best interest of the patient. In many cases in which a patient has suffered a devastating injury that leaves him or her unable to breathe spontaneously (that is, without external assistance), there is little chance that use of a ventilator will lead to much improvement in the patient's condition. The reason for this is that an inability to breathe spontaneously is often the result of a very serious injury to the brain. Saving a patient from death after such an injury turns out, in many cases, to be an ambiguous sort of success. This ambiguity often leads physicians and patients' loved ones to decide that death should be allowed to come even when the ventilator is capable of putting it off for a time.[1]

B. "Coma Dépassé"—Beyond Coma

With the introduction of the ventilator, however, a different sort of problem emerged as well. Some brain-injured patients, dependent on the ventilator to breathe, turn out to be definitively more incapacitated than others who at first seem to be in a similar state. In 1959, French neurologists Pierre Mollaret and Maurice Goullon characterized this condition of maximal incapacitation. The label they provided for it was *coma dépassé*, or "beyond coma."[2]

At the same time, other physicians were discovering the same clinical facts about some of their own patients. In response, many medical experts concluded that what the ventilator accomplishes in these cases is very different from what it accomplishes in cases in which the patient is less incapacitated. In their judgment, a patient who is "beyond coma" is not being kept *barely alive* by the machine but, rather, is *already dead*. The machine is, in essence, ventilating a corpse—albeit one that in many ways does not look like a corpse. Today, other terms are used in place of *coma dépassé*, including the confusing and misleading term "brain death." The question of terminology will be explored more fully in Chapter Two.

Those who understood the *coma dépassé* condition in this way distinguished, therefore, two groups of brain-injured, ventilator-dependent individuals. Members of one group of patients are already dead and should therefore be removed from the ventilator. The apparent signs of life that remain—a beating heart, warm skin, and minimal, if any, signs of bodily decay—are a sort of mask that hides from plain sight the fact that the biological organism has ceased to function as such. Members of the other group of patients are *not* already dead. For them—but not for the first group—an ethical dilemma arises as to whether further medical treatment is futile and should be discontinued, thus allowing them to die.

C. The Harvard Committee and the President's Commission

The point of view that accepts this distinction has become the dominant one in most parts of the world, including the United

States. In 1968, a physician-led committee at Harvard Medical School, in an influential paper entitled "A Definition of Irreversible Coma," concluded that patients who meet the diagnostic criteria for a certain type of severe brain injury may be pronounced dead before the heart stops beating.[3] In the 1970s, various state legislatures and courts acted to turn this "medical consensus" into a legally recognized standard for determining death.[*] Not all states took such action; those that did formulated the new brain-based physiological standard and its relation to the more traditional cardiopulmonary standard in often significantly different ways. In 1981, the President's Commission for the Study of Ethical Problems in Medicine and Biomedical and Behavioral Research (hereinafter "the President's Commission") published *Defining Death: Medical, Legal and Ethical Issues in the Determination of Death*. In this landmark report, the President's Commission proposed a uniform statute for determining death by the application of two alternative physiological standards: (1) "irreversible cessation of circulatory and respiratory functions" and (2) "irreversible cessation of all functions of the entire brain, including the brainstem."[4]

The text accompanying the proposed uniform statute clarified the relationship between the two alternative standards. It said that in almost all cases of human death the traditional standard (i.e., irreversible cessation of circulatory and respiratory functions) should be used, as it always had been. Only in rare cases in which mechanical ventilation is used to support the breathing of a severely brain-injured individual—one who meets criteria similar to those laid out

---

[*] Whether it truly was a consensus is a matter of historical debate. Certainly there were some prominent physicians and others who did not share the Harvard committee's confidence that those who were properly diagnosed with "brain death" (or "irreversible coma," as the 1968 report called it) were dead as human beings. Some discussion of this issue can be found in M. S. Pernick, "Back from the Grave: Recurring Controversies over Defining and Diagnosing Death in History," in *Death: Beyond Whole Brain Criteria*, ed. R. Zaner (The Netherlands: Kluwer Academic Publishers, 1988), 17-74; and M. S. Pernick, "Brain Death in a Cultural Context: The Reconstruction of Death, 1967-1981," in *The Definition of Death: Contemporary Controversies*, ed. S. J. Youngner, R. M. Arnold, and R. Schapiro (Baltimore: The Johns Hopkins University Press, 1999): 3-33.

by the Harvard committee—should a brain-based standard be employed.

According to the President's Commission, these latter cases require a non-traditional standard because circulatory and respiratory functions cannot and should not be considered signs of continued life if they are supported *technologically*. The Commission proposed a useful metaphor for the problem: recognizing death is like looking into a room to see if someone is there. When the window that one usually peers through is obscured—when the curtain is drawn—one should make every effort to find another window. In the case at hand, the "curtain is drawn" by the use of the ventilator to support breathing and (indirectly) circulation. According to the President's Commission, the neurological standard of irreversible loss of whole brain function—the *coma dépassé* or "brain death" diagnosis—is a second window on the same, biologically real phenomenon of human death. Such a standard is needed only when the traditional standard cannot be used—only when the curtain is drawn on the first window do we need to look through the second.

The President's Commission's model statute was endorsed by the American Medical Association (AMA), the American Bar Association (ABA), and the National Conference of Commissioners on Uniform State Laws (NCCUSL). The NCCUSL published this statute under the name "Uniform Determination of Death Act" (UDDA) and worked to get it passed in all of the states and jurisdictions of the United States. The key section of the Act, Section One, reads as follows:

> §1. [Determination of Death]. An individual who has sustained either (1) irreversible cessation of circulatory and respiratory functions, or (2) irreversible cessation of all functions of the entire brain, including the brain stem, is dead. A determination of death must be made in accordance with accepted medical standards.[5]

Through the NCCUSL's efforts, a significant increase in uniformity has been achieved. Not all U.S. jurisdictions have adopted the exact language of the UDDA, but all of them, without exception, have some form of legal recognition for a brain-based standard of death.[*] This recognition allows physicians to declare an individual who is dependent on a ventilator dead before the cessation of heartbeat and respiration *if* results indicating the *coma dépassé* or "brain death" condition are obtained upon neurological examination.

The consensus position for using a neurological standard to determine death in the United States may be stated in this way: "Whole brain death"—but no other sort of injury that leaves circulation and respiration intact—is an appropriate standard for determining the death of a human being.

D. The Contemporary Controversy

Today, however, the consensus position is subject to a number of persistent concerns and novel criticisms. There remains considerable public confusion, both about the meaning of the term "brain dead" and about its relation to the death of a human being. There is persistent dissent by some clinicians, philosophers, and other critical observers who have never been convinced that "brain death" is, indeed, the death of the human being. There are, as well, pressures against insisting that declaring death, or at least "organ donation eligibility," requires the irreversible loss of function in the whole brain. And, perhaps most important, there are critics who have published evidence of ongoing integrated bodily activities in some persons meeting the criteria of "whole brain death" and who have claimed that this evidence invalidates the rationale for today's consensus position. These challenges invite—indeed, they necessitate— a re-examination of the neurological standard enshrined in law and medical practice. In this report, the President's Council on Bioethics offers such a re-examination.

---

[*] Forty-five U.S. jurisdictions have adopted a determination of death act that is either identical to, or shares basic elements with, the UDDA. For details, see H. R. Beresford, "Legal Aspects of Brain Death," in *Brain Death*, ed. E. F. Wijdicks (Philadelphia: Lippincott Williams & Wilkins, 2001). A few states have no determination of death statute, but rely instead on precedent-setting court cases, some of which cite the UDDA in their decisions.

II. The Aims and Rationale of This Report

A. *Educating the Public*

One aim of this report is to illuminate for the American public and its policymakers the complexities inherent in the current legal and medical understanding of death. Certain questions emerge immediately: What is "whole brain death"? How do clinicians determine that such a condition is present in a given patient? What pathophysiological and prognostic facts about the condition support the judgment that "whole brain death" is more than just another case of human injury—that it is, rather, the death of the human being? How can the confusions engendered by the term "brain death" be dispelled?

B. *Addressing Challenges to the Neurological Standard*

Another aim of this report is to address various challenges to the prevailing view that have emerged over the years. In truth, the clinical and pathophysiological facts about the "whole brain death" condition are better understood today than they were in 1968 or 1981. This improved understanding of the facts invites a re-examination of a standard that crucially depends, for its validity, on those facts. Some critics who have undertaken this work of re-examination have concluded that the neurological standard for death is not justifiable—that, in light of what we now know, only the traditional signs of death are adequate for confidently determining that a human being has made the transition from living body to corpse. Such a conclusion is shared also by a minority that has long held itself apart from the emerging consensus, doubting whether any patient who continues to breathe and whose blood circulates—even with technological help—can confidently be judged *already dead*. Thus, in this report, the President's Council also reconsiders the philosophical adequacy of the prevailing view on "brain death."

C. Clarifying the Troubled Relationship Between Determining Death and Procuring Organs

One more critical impetus for this inquiry must be mentioned and explored. As previously noted, the "whole brain death" standard for determining death has also been challenged by critics interested in increasing the supply of organs for transplantation. Additional background will be helpful in understanding the nature of this challenge.[*]

A human being whose death has been determined according to a neurological standard is the ideal source of transplantable organs. The reason for this is straightforward: with artificial support of respiration and circulation, blood continues to circulate through the body, thereby maintaining the vitality of organs targeted for surgical removal and thus optimizing their utility for their eventual recipients. If surgeons wait for the more traditional signs of death, the organs endure a period of "warm ischemia" during which they are deprived of nourishing blood and oxygen. While it is possible to procure some organs under these circumstances, concerns about ischemic damage make the heart-beating, "brain-dead" donor the preferred source of organs.[†]

The advantage of the "heart-beating cadaver" for transplantation was not missed, of course, by the pioneering physicians and policymakers who advocated early on for the now widely accepted

---

[*] A full treatment of the history, practice, and ethics of organ transplantation can be found in the Council's report on that subject, published as a companion volume to this report. The discussion here covers only those facts most relevant to the "determination of death" topic.

[†] Chapter Six discusses procurement of organs (e.g., kidneys, lungs, livers, hearts, pancreata, and intestines) from donors whose death has been determined based on the cessation of circulatory and respiratory function. Also, the remarks here do not pertain to the procurement of what is commonly referred to as "tissue" (as opposed to organs) from a cadaver. In this context, tissue refers to skin, bones, heart valves, corneas, tendons, and veins—all parts of the body that can be taken from a cadaver and put to medical use for another human being. These parts can be taken hours after the heart has stopped beating.

neurological standard. The Harvard committee, for instance, mentioned avoiding "controversy in obtaining organs for transplantation" as one of two primary practical goods that would come from the new understanding of death.*

After the Harvard committee released its report, a group of prominent physicians, philosophers, and bioethicists known as the "Task Force on Death and Dying of the Institute of Society, Ethics and the Life Sciences" (hereinafter "the Task Force") published an appraisal of the new standard for determining death. In that paper, the group made it clear that, although the conclusions regarding a neurological standard would certainly have the effect of creating "available organ sources," the neurological standard was not designed solely to accomplish that end.[6] It should be noted that there were some who did not accept the Task Force's judgment and suspected that the movement for a brain-based death standard was driven by the need for transplantable organs.

Nonetheless, the Task Force's clarification has largely set the tone for all subsequent debate: The question of whether a human being in the difficult-to-judge state of "brain death" is alive or dead should be answered on its own terms, not with an eye to the practical effects that a new standard for determining death might have. In other words, society must first decide how to understand the condition of ventilator-dependent patients who have suffered the most debilitating kind of brain injury: Are these individuals dead? Can we *know* that they are dead with the requisite amount of certainty to act accordingly? Only after these questions have been answered can the matter of eligibility for organ procurement be addressed.

The Council's inquiry into controversies surrounding the determination of death is firmly situated in this tradition. The central

---

* The other good it mentioned was relieving the burden on families and caregivers of providing invasive, expensive, and—crucially—*futile* medical treatment. Today, this problem is less acute since patients and their surrogate decision makers have a greater degree of control over decisions to remove interventions. Doing so does not rely in any way on deciding that the patient is *already dead*.

question addressed by the Council is, *Does a diagnosis of "whole brain death" mean that the human being is dead?* That is to say, the central question is not, *Does a diagnosis of "whole brain death" mean that the human being is eligible to be a heart-beating organ donor?*

Even so, it would be unwise to take up the issue of the "whole brain" neurological standard for death without some acknowledgment of the pivotal role that the standard plays in transplantation medicine. In its companion inquiry into the ethics of organ transplantation, the Council examines various policy proposals offered as solutions to the growing gap between the need for and the supply of human organs. It also considers, in particular, ongoing debates about the ethics of procuring organs from individuals with various degrees of neurological injury, including patients in persistent vegetative states. For this reason, some preliminary discussion of how the determination of death fits into the larger picture of organ procurement is warranted.

Organs can be procured from either the living or the dead, but the living donor can only ethically give organs whose removal will not adversely affect his or her ability to live in a relatively healthy state. *All* organs and types of tissue that are useful for transplant can be taken from the deceased, but only if valid consent has been obtained.* To count as "deceased," an individual must meet one of the two standards described in the UDDA. In the majority of cases, the standard used to declare death prior to organ procurement is the neurological standard; to meet this standard, the patient-donor must be conclusively diagnosed with the condition known as "whole brain death."†

---

* For more information on consent policies, see D. Wendler and N. Dickert, "The Consent Process for Cadaveric Organ Procurement: How Does It Work? How Can It Be Improved?" *JAMA* 285, no. 3 (2001); and Chapter Three of the Council's report on organ transplantation.

† Cases where organ procurement occurs after a declaration of death by the cardio-pulmonary standard are discussed in detail in Chapter Six.

Some proponents of organ transplantation argue that these ethical constraints restrict access to the goods that transplantation makes possible: improved health for recipients and the opportunity for generous acts by donors and families in the face of loss and grief. To increase the supply of organs, they argue, more leeway should be given to individuals and families to choose organ donation when a human being is, as the law is now construed, *near* death—that is, *before* the strict neurological standard for death has been met.

Reforming the practice of organ donation and procurement to make more organs available could take two forms: (1) loosening the standard for determining death, or (2) abandoning what is known as the "dead donor rule"—the requirement that an individual be "really dead" in order to be a heart-beating donor of vital organs.

With the first option, some individuals with brain injuries less severe than "whole brain death" would also be regarded as dead. Some advocates of this measure argue that a person is dead when certain higher brain functions (or mental capacities) are gone. They would endorse changing the legal/medical definition of death to encompass this group and, still following the mandate of the "dead donor rule," allow them to serve as heart-beating organ donors.[7]

The second option would leave the legal/medical definition of death as it stands (or even change it to require cessation of circulation), but would allow the removal of organs from brain-injured patients who are very close to death (but not yet dead). In this revised scheme, clear consent for organ removal—which would occur before death—would be required. Proponents of the second option seek to avoid the philosophical tangles of deciding whether a neurological standard for death is justified without losing the benefits that come from removing organs from heart-beating patients.[8]

In this report, the Council will contend that arguments for both reform options are unconvincing. As regards the first option, the Council maintains that there is no "looser standard of death" that can stand up to biological and philosophical scrutiny. Arguments that have been made in support of a looser standard are based on an impoverished view of what it is to be a human being. The Council's position on this is elaborated in Chapter Four.

As for the second reform option, that is, abandoning the "dead donor rule" as a guide for practice—the Council believes this is not ethically justifiable. If indeed it is the case that there is no solid scientific or philosophical rationale for the current "whole brain standard," then the only ethical course is to stop procuring organs from heart-beating individuals. Organ transplantation could continue, but with exclusive reliance on donors whose death is determined by the cardiopulmonary standard under a controlled DCD protocol (see Chapter Six for details). In the majority view of the Council, such a step is not necessary, however, since today's "whole brain standard" is, in fact, conceptually sound.

III. The Organization of This Report

The discussion thus far has described the current state of the theory and the practice of determining death using a neurological standard. A few important points warrant repeated emphasis: First, the central question of this report is, *Are patients diagnosed with "whole brain death" dead as human beings?* A related, secondary question is, *How should new empirical findings about "whole brain death" be interpreted?*

Chapter Two of this report offers a critique of the term "brain death" as a description of the clinical condition of the patients whose status as living or dead is at the center of debate. The term is problematic. Whether patients in this condition are, in fact, dead, is the central uncertainty addressed by this report; therefore, a term employing the word "death"—as "brain death" or "whole brain death" does—is prejudicial to the aims of an open inquiry. With this concern in mind, we propose the term "total brain failure" for the *clinical diagnosis* that underlies the current neurological standard.

Chapter Three presents a thorough discussion of the clinical and pathophysiological details that must be understood in order to evaluate the validity of a neurological standard for determining death. This chapter has five main parts. Part I is an account of the "vital functions" of breathing and circulation, with an emphasis on the role of the central nervous system in their operation. The chapter then turns to the clinical state, "total brain failure," that is, the condition typically referred to as "whole brain death." In Part II, this clinical state is examined from the standpoint of diagnostics: How can clinicians recognize that an injured individual is, indeed, properly diagnosed with this condition? In Part III, the condition is analyzed from the standpoint of pathophysiology: What is going on in the brain and body of a patient with a diagnosis that meets the criteria of "total brain failure"? In Part IV, empirical findings about the condition that have emerged in recent years are explored. These are findings that some consider damaging to the rationale for the "whole brain death" standard. The fifth part of Chapter Three is a comparison of total brain failure with a state of brain injury with which it is often confused—the persistent vegetative state or PVS.

Chapter Four develops in detail two opposing positions on the central question of the report, *Are individuals diagnosed with total brain failure—more generally known as "whole brain death"—really dead as human beings?* The first of these takes a principled, agnostic posture: We cannot know with certainty that patients with total brain failure are dead or alive and, as a result, such patients should be regarded as living until their hearts stop. The second position in Chapter Four affirms the current neurological standard, but develops an argument for it based on different philosophical premises than those that have become commonplace.

In Chapter Five, we examine the implications for policy and practice of each of the positions described in Chapter Four. We do so with a concern both for the needs of organ transplantation and the need to respect the dignity of patients at the end of life.

Chapter Six explores the practice of controlled DCD. This increasingly common practice in U.S. hospitals provides a family with the opportunity to donate the vital organs of a terminally injured loved one after he or she dies. If the family agrees to donation, then the death of a loved one is monitored in a controlled setting that allows the transplant team to retrieve the organs from the donor as soon as the heart stops. Death is determined by the cardiopulmonary standard, but the timing of the determination is dictated by the requirements of successful organ procurement. For this reason, there can be unsettling ambiguities in the line between life and death with controlled DCD—and thus ethical concerns that merit thoughtful consideration. In Chapter Six, we briefly explore these concerns, which the Council also examines in detail in its report on the ethics of organ transplantation.

In the final chapter, Chapter Seven, we summarize the conclusions of the Council's inquiry into current controversies in the determination of death, taking note of its discussions of ethical concerns in controlled DCD, but focusing on its debate about the biological and philosophical justification of the neurological standard.

⋘⋙

ENDNOTES

[1] For studies on how often this occurs, see T. J. Prendergast and J. M. Luce, "Increasing Incidence of Withholding and Withdrawal of Life Support from the Critically Ill," *Am J Respir Crit Care Med* 155, no. 1 (1997): 15-20; and S. P. Keenan et al., "A Retrospective Review of a Large Cohort of Patients Undergoing the Process of Withholding or Withdrawal of Life Support," *Crit Care Med* 25, no. 8 (1997): 1324-31.

[2] P. Mollaret and M. Goulon, "Le Coma Dépassé," *Rev Neurol (Paris)* 101 (1959): 3-15. For a survey of the early neurological literature regarding this subgroup of ventilator-dependent patients, see M. N. Diringer and E. F. Wijdicks, "Brain Death in Historical Perspective," in *Brain Death*, ed. E. F. Wijdicks (Philadelphia: Lippincott Williams & Wilkins, 2001): 5-27; E. F. Wijdicks, "The Neurologist and Harvard Criteria for Brain Death," *Neurology* 61, no. 7 (2003): 970-6; C. Machado, "The First Organ Transplant from a Brain-Dead Donor," *Neurology* 64, no. 11 (2005): 1938-42; and C. Machado et al., "The Concept of Brain Death Did Not Evolve to Benefit Organ Transplants," *J Med Ethics* 33, no. 4 (2007): 197-200.

[3] Ad Hoc Committee of the Harvard Medical School to Examine the Definition of Brain Death, "A Definition of Irreversible Coma," *JAMA* 205, no. 6 (1968): 337-40.

[4] President's Commission for the Study of Ethical Problems in Medicine and Biomedical and Behavioral Research, *Defining Death: Medical, Legal and Ethical Issues in the Determination of Death,* (Washington, D.C.: Government Printing Office, 1981). Available online at http://www.bioethics.gov/reports/past_commissions/defining_death.pdf (accessed Oct. 22, 2008).

[5] The complete text of the act is available online at http://www.law.upenn.edu/bll/archives/ulc/fnact99/1980s/udda80.htm. (accessed Sept. 26, 2008).

[6] Institute of Society, Ethics, and the Life Sciences, Task Force on Death and Dying, "Refinements in Criteria for the Determination of Death: An Appraisal," *JAMA* 221, no. 1 (1972): 48-53.

[7] See, for instance, K. G. Gervais, *Redefining Death* (New Haven: Yale University Press, 1986); R. M. Veatch, "The Death of Whole-Brain Death: The Plague of the Disaggregators, Somaticists, and Mentalists," *J Med Philos* 30, no. 4 (2005): 353-78; and J. P. Lizza, *Persons, Humanity, and the Definition of Death* (Baltimore, Md.: Johns Hopkins University Press, 2006).

[8] See, for instance, R. M. Arnold and S. J. Youngner, "The Dead Donor Rule: Should We Stretch It, Bend It, or Abandon It?" *Kennedy Inst Ethics J* 3, no. 2 (1993): 263-78; N. Fost, "Reconsidering the Dead Donor Rule: Is It Important That Organ Donors Be Dead?" *Kennedy Inst Ethics J* 14, no. 3 (2004): 249-60; and R. D. Truog, "Brain Death—Too Flawed to Endure, Too Ingrained to Abandon," *J Law Med Ethics* 35, no. 2 (2007): 273-81. The conceptual case for "eligibility for donation without knowledge of death" was described earlier in R. S. Morison, "Death: Process or Event?" *Science* 173, no. 998 (1971): 694-8; R. B. Dworkin, "Death in Context," *Indiana Law J* 48, no. 4 (1973): 623-39; and A. Halevy and B. Brody, "Brain Death: Reconciling Definitions, Criteria, and Tests," *Ann Intern Med* 119, no. 6 (1993): 519-25.

CHAPTER TWO

TERMINOLOGY

Although commonly used to identify the neurological standard for determining death, the term "brain death" is highly problematic. Three difficulties, in particular, are noteworthy.

First, the term "brain death" implies that there is more than one kind of death. This is a serious error, perpetuated by such statements as "the patient became brain dead at 3:00 a.m. on Thursday and died two days later." Whatever difficulties there might be in knowing whether death has occurred, it must be kept in mind that there is only one *real* phenomenon of death. Death is the transition from being a living, mortal organism to being something that, though dead, retains a physical continuity with the once-living organism. Some will argue that such a transition does not occur instantaneously or that there are cases in which there is no way to *know* if the transition has, in fact, occurred. But, problems of "knowing" aside, there is only one real phenomenon that clinicians and families struggle to recognize.

Second, the term "brain death" implies that death is a state of the cells and tissues constituting the brain. In fact, what is directly at issue is the living or dead status of the human individual, not the individual's brain. In other contexts, it may be useful to talk about the death of *parts* of the body—the death of a cell, for example, or the "death" (irreversible failure) of an organ, such as a kidney or a liver. In current law and medical practice, the condition that warrants a determination of death using the neurological standard is *not* the "death of the brain" in this sense.

17

For this reason, evidence of continued activity of the pituitary gland, or of similar residual brain tissue function in patients diagnosed with "brain death," is not decisive in determining whether these patients are living or dead.* The question is not, *Has the whole brain died?* The question is, *Has the human being died?* This criticism can be leveled perhaps even more sharply at the commonly employed phrase "whole brain death," which, if taken literally, implies that every part of the brain must be non-functional for the diagnosis to be made. In reality, and somewhat at odds with the exact wording of the UDDA, "*all* functions of the entire brain" do not have to be extinguished in order to meet the neurological standard under the current application of the law to medical practice. In Chapter Four, we take up the question, "On what grounds might we judge the persistence of certain functions (e.g., ADH secretion by the pituitary gland) to be less important than other functions (e.g., spontaneous breathing)?"

Third, death itself is not a diagnosis; that is, the phenomenon of death and the selection of the appropriate standard for determining it are not strictly medical or technical matters. Thus, any term chosen as a label for a *medical* diagnosis should not contain the word "death." It is not death that is diagnosed but rather a clinical state or condition made evident by certain ascertainable signs. Calling the condition of the patient who meets a set of diagnostic tests "brain death" begs the question of whether this condition does or does not warrant a determination that the patient has died. What is needed is a separate, non-prejudicial name for the condition that describes the state of the patient: a name that does not, by its use, commit one to any judgment about whether the death of the human being has occurred.

Other commentators over the years have noted similar difficulties with the term "brain death." In response, various terms have been suggested to replace it as the name for the clinical diagnosis. The

---

* This evidence is discussed more completely in Part III of Chapter Three.

table below compiles some of these terms, along with references to their respective sources in the scholarly literature.

Table 1: Different Terms for One Clinical State

Term	*Sources*
(Whole/Total) Brain Death	Terms most commonly used today
Total Brain Failure	Preferred term of this report
Coma Dépassé ("Beyond Coma")	Mollaret and Goulon, 1959
Irreversible Coma	Harvard committee, 1968
(Total) Brain Infarction	Ingvar, 1971[1]; Shewmon, 1997[2]
Irreversible Apneic Coma	Zamperetti, et al., 2004[3]
Brain Arrest	Shemie, et al., 2006[4]

Each term has advantages and disadvantages. Although the choice of an appropriate term is important, it is more crucial to maintain a distinction between naming the medical diagnosis of a condition and declaring an individual dead on the basis of that medical diagnosis. In this report, we will employ the term "total brain failure" for the medical diagnosis. The precise meaning of "total" in this composite term is discussed in Chapter Three. Here, at the outset, we emphasize that total brain failure is, by definition, an *irreversible* condition. Thus, to be more explicit one could employ the term, "total and irreversible brain failure." We will use the more familiar terms, "brain death" or "whole brain death," when such use is warranted by the specific context, for example, in describing the history of the concept or in referencing works by others who themselves use these more familiar terms.

Because there is no perfect term, the choice of one is necessarily somewhat arbitrary. Nonetheless, an exploration of the strengths and weaknesses of the different terms can be useful in understanding the relevant clinical and pathophysiological facts. This will become clearer in Chapter Three, where we assume different perspectives on the clinical condition that is at the center of the debate.

ENDNOTES

[1] D. H. Ingvar, "Brain Death—Total Brain Infarction," *Acta Anaesthesiol Scand Suppl* 45 (1971): 129-40.

[2] D. A. Shewmon, "Recovery from 'Brain Death': A Neurologist's Apologia," *Linacre Q* 64, no. 1 (1997): 30-96.

[3] N. Zamperetti. et al., "Irreversible Apnoeic Coma 35 Years Later. Towards a More Rigorous Definition of Brain Death?" *Intensive Care Med* 30, no. 9 (2004): 1715-22.

[4] S. D. Shemie, et al., "Severe Brain Injury to Neurological Determination of Death: Canadian Forum Recommendations," *CMAJ* 174, no. 6 (2006): S1-13.

CHAPTER THREE

THE CLINICAL PRESENTATION AND PATHOPHYSIOLOGY OF TOTAL BRAIN FAILURE

B efore we engage the central question—*Is a human being diagnosed with total brain failure dead?*—we need to recount some of the more salient aspects of the clinical presentation and underlying pathophysiology of total brain failure. We begin with a description of the functions of circulation and respiration. Under the usual circumstances, the presence of these processes in a body is a sure sign of life. Understanding how breathing and circulation operate in normal circumstances will illuminate why this is so—why, that is, these are aptly called "vital functions."

In patients who are diagnosed with total brain failure and, on this basis, are declared dead, these vital functions are dependent on external support from the ventilator. To defenders of today's neurological standard, this means that these *apparent* signs of life are, in fact, artifacts of the technological support—they conceal the fact that death has already occurred. To evaluate this argument, the basic facts of *technological support for these vital functions* must be made clear. This clarity can only be achieved if the interrelatedness of the three body systems involved in breathing and circulation is understood. The three systems are:

1. The heart and circulatory system.
2. The lungs and respiratory system.
3. The central nervous system and, in particular, the centers involved in breathing.

After describing these vital functions and clarifying the nature of technological support for these functions in Part I, we explain why a patient who has the loss of the ability to breathe is not necessarily dead. In Part II, we take up the diagnosis of total brain failure and explain how patients with this diagnosis are distinguished from those with less serious forms of neurological injury. In Part III, we turn to the pathophysiology of total brain failure, that is, to the processes that unfold with this condition at the level of brain tissues and cells. In Part IV, we address two types of medical findings that have led some to question the suitability of total brain failure as a clinically and ethically valid standard for assessing death. In Part V, we compare total brain failure with the vegetative state and survey recent discussions of consciousness and functional states of the human brain.

I. The "Vital Functions" in Health and After Brain Injury

The pathophysiological processes that eventually end in the mortal condition we are calling total brain failure engage not only the central nervous system but also the circulatory and respiratory systems of the human body. In this account of these systems and the vital functions that they make possible—and that eventually fail with total brain failure—we begin with respiration.

A. Oxygen In, Carbon Dioxide Out

Under usual circumstances, an adult human being inhales and exhales twelve to twenty times per minute. Each inhalation is effected by a contraction of muscles in the thorax or chest cavity, the most important of which is the diaphragm. These muscles can collectively be termed the "muscles of respiration" (See Figure 1).

The contraction of these muscles causes the lungs to expand and the body to take in air from the surrounding atmosphere. This air enters through the nose and mouth and travels to the lungs via the respiratory tree. At the terminal end of this tree with its multiple branches are the pulmonary alveoli, which are small spherical air sacs surrounded by tiny blood vessels (See Figure 2). The walls of the alveoli are extremely thin, formed to facilitate diffusion of gases between the sacs and the blood vessels (See Figure 3).

Figure 1: The Muscles Involved in Respiration

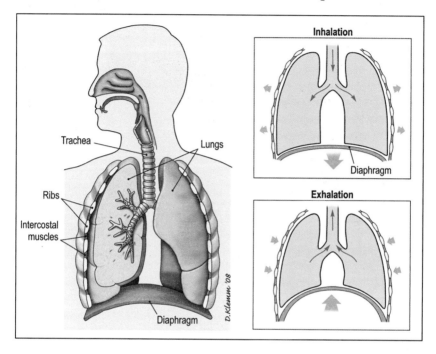

Figure 2: The Respiratory Tree and Alveoli

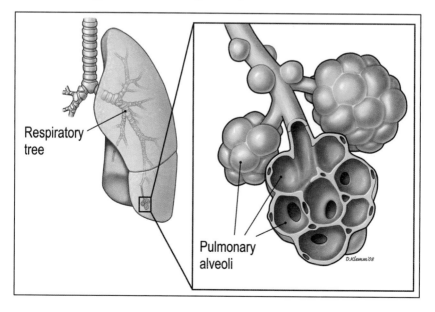

Figure 3: Detail of Alveoli

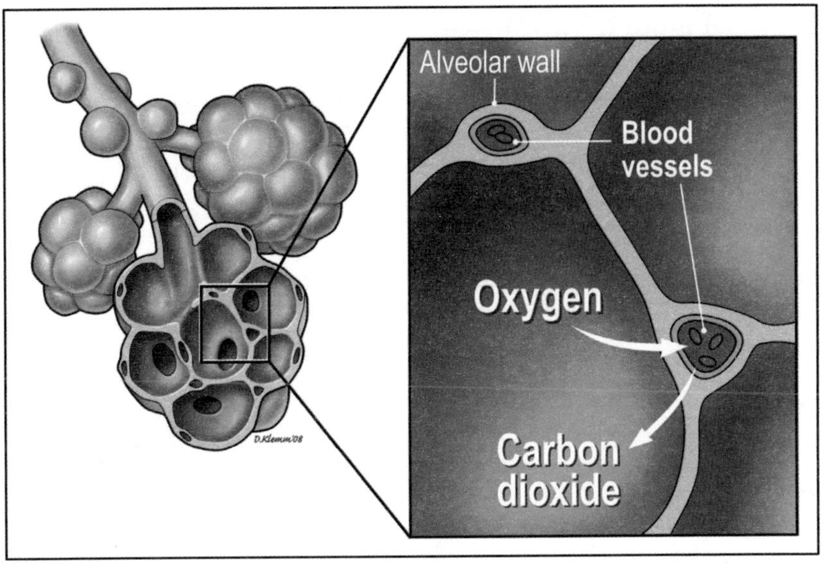

To *inhale* is to bring air to these terminal nodes where oxygen from the atmospheric air is able to move into the blood. Oxygen is critical to the ongoing metabolic work of the millions of cells in the body. Without a continuous supply of oxygen, brought into the body through inhalations and transported to the tissues by circulating blood, the body's cells, tissues, and organs would cease to function.

Exhaling is just as critical to the life of a human being or other animal organism. When the cells of the body perform their work—metabolic and otherwise—they produce waste products, notably carbon dioxide (CO_2). This CO_2 is carried away from the cells by the blood that returns to the heart and lungs. In the same act of exchange by diffusion that brings oxygen *in* at the alveoli, CO_2 diffuses *out* from blood to the alveolar cavity (See Figure 3). From the alveolar cavity, air that is now rich in CO_2 moves back up the respiratory tree and out into the surrounding atmosphere. This expulsion or exhalation of carbon dioxide is brought about, mechanically, by the relaxation of the muscles of respiration and the subsequent shrinking of the cavities of the lungs. Again, it is vital to the organism as a whole that this removal of CO_2 from the body be continually accomplished.

Thus, inhaling and exhaling—the process of breathing—facilitate a critical exchange between the organism and the world. To put it in the simplest of terms: the exchange is one of oxygen in and carbon dioxide out, and the purpose of the exchange is to fuel the cellular processes of metabolism with oxygen and to rid the body of the waste products of those processes. The mechanism of the exchange includes the contraction and the relaxation of the muscles of respiration and the diffusion of gases into the blood across the lining of the tiny alveoli.

B. The Role of the Central Nervous System and Ventilator Support

For many years it was not well understood that the Central Nervous System (CNS), comprising the brain and the spinal cord, plays a crucial role in maintaining an organism's vital functions. To understand that role, one might begin by pondering how it is that the muscles of respiration "know" when to contract. Does this contraction happen in an automatic, periodic fashion or does it happen upon receiving some *signal* from the body's CNS? The answer is this: the contraction of the muscles of respiration is brought about by a signal sent from the respiratory center of the CNS. That center is located at the base of the brainstem,[*] in a structure known as the medulla oblongata (The anatomical references in this and the ensuing discussion are illustrated in Figure 4 on page 26.)

When sensors in the respiratory center detect a relatively high level of CO_2 in the blood, a signal is sent to the muscles of respiration, spurring them to contract. Each of the twelve to twenty inhalations per minute, then, is the body's response to the accumulation of the waste products of metabolism; for life to continue, the CO_2 must be expelled and new oxygen must be brought in.

---

[*] On the functions of the brainstem, see Part II below.

Other parts of the CNS can also be involved in signaling the muscles of respiration to contract so that oxygen-rich air will be inhaled. In what is called "conscious breathing," a human being can deliberately control the depth and pace of breathing, during which time other parts of the brain are involved in controlling the muscles of respiration. Changes in the depth and pace of breathing can also be brought about without conscious effort: the rate of breathing will quicken, for example, during physical exercise or in response to a "fight or flight" situation. These changes are directed by changing metabolic needs (current or anticipated) throughout the body's organs and tissues.

Figure 4: The Brain and Brainstem, with Major Divisions

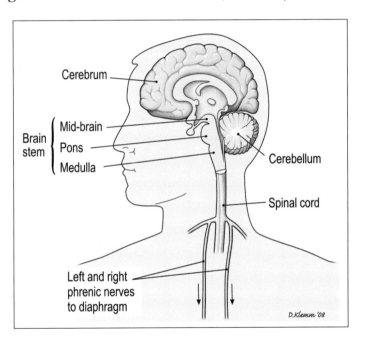

For the purposes of our inquiry, the crucial fact about the mechanics of breathing is this: When the brainstem's respiratory centers are incapacitated, the organism will not make or display any respiratory effort. The chest will remain absolutely still and the body's need for oxygen will go unanswered. If the death of the organism is to be prevented, some external "driver" of the breathing process—a mechanical ventilator—must be used.*

The mechanical ventilator works by increasing and decreasing the pressure in the lung cavities so that oxygen-rich atmospheric air will travel down and CO_2-rich air will travel back up the respiratory tree. Gas exchange in the lungs is then possible, although an external substitute for the patient's own respiratory effort cannot manage this exchange (and thus maintain ideal blood-gas levels) as effectively as the body free of injury can. The exchange of gases that the ventilator sustains will be of no benefit to the patient unless the blood is kept moving as well. Incoming oxygen must be transported to the tissues that need it, and accumulating carbon dioxide must be removed to the lungs for expulsion from the body. In other words, the ventilator will help the patient only if another vital organ system is operational, comprising the heart, working as a pump, and the conveying network of arteries, veins, and capillaries.

C. Circulation of Blood

The action of the circulatory system is analogous to the action of the external respiratory system.[†] Each system acts to maintain the continuous motion of a fluid substance that fuels the metabolic work of the organism as a whole. The fluid substance is *air* in respi-

---

* There is another sort of situation in which a ventilator is required to support vital functions: The respiratory center in the brain can be functional while the muscles of respiration themselves are paralyzed. This was the case for polio patients in the mid-20th century who were the first wide-scale recipients of ventilatory treatment in the form of cumbersome iron lung machines (i.e., negative pressure ventilators). Here, one could say, the CNS signal to take action is being sent, but it is falling on "deaf ears." Alternatively, one may say that the *drive* to breathe is present but the ability to turn that drive into action is absent. For many polio patients, the paralysis subsided when the virus was defeated and, as a result, normal breathing resumed.

† The *external* respiratory system is the part of the respiratory system that engages the organism with the outside world. By contrast, the *internal* respiratory system functions at the cellular level to assimilate oxygen from the bloodstream and deposit CO_2 back into the bloodstream.

ration and *blood* in circulation. Furthermore, in both respiration and circulation, the mechanism of action is the periodic contraction of muscle—the heart muscle in circulation, the muscles of respiration in breathing.*

There are important differences, however, between the circulatory work of moving blood and the respiratory work of moving air in the body. The movement of blood occurs only within the body, whereas the movement of air is an exchange between the body and the surrounding atmosphere. This point will be important to the discussion of "Position Two" in Chapter Four. Another difference, more relevant to the present explanation of external support of vital systems, is the fact that there is no part of the CNS that is *absolutely indispensable* for heart contractions in the way that the respiratory center in the brainstem is absolutely indispensable for the muscular contractions involved in breathing.

Again, in healthy circumstances, stimuli from the CNS will alter the rate and strength of contractions: the heart rate will change in response to danger, excitement, or other stimuli. But even when there is no stimulus whatsoever from the CNS, the heart can continue to beat. This property of the heart, known as its "inherent rhythmicity," has been demonstrated dramatically by experiments in which an animal's heart is taken out of its body and stimulated to begin beating rhythmically again. It is also demonstrated by the heartbeat of an embryo, which begins before the CNS has developed.

---

* This description is incomplete insofar as it suggests that the heart is the only active part of the circulatory system. In fact, the *vessels* of circulation, far from being rigid "plumbing lines" that passively convey blood pumped by the heart, are living tissues that undergo changes (some driven by the CNS) to maintain an appropriate blood pressure. Patients who are receiving ventilatory support often must also be given drugs (e.g., pressors) to help keep the blood pressure in a healthy range.

D. Ventilator Support and Determination of Death

What, then, does it mean to say that the ventilator "externally sup-ports the vital functions of breathing and circulation?" It means that, in the place of the organism's effort to breathe, stimulated by the respiratory centers of the CNS, an external device moves the lungs and facilitates the inflow and outflow of needed air. This al-lows the heart muscle to continue to function, because its cells, like all other cells in the body, need oxygen to stay alive. The defense of the neurological standard for determining death begins with these observations: respiratory motion supported in this way is not in it-self a "sign of life." It is, rather, an artifact of technological intervention. Nor is a beating heart, in these circumstances, a "sign of life." It is, instead, merely the continuation of an automatic proc-ess that would quickly cease if the ventilator were withdrawn. The defense of the neurological standard *begins* with these points, but it does not rest its case there. The loss of the ability to breathe on one's own is not a sufficient condition for declaring that an individ-ual has died. Two other conditions are necessary: (1) other functions indicative of life must be lost, and (2) these functional losses must be *irreversible*. Each of these conditions warrants further explanation.

Any doubt that the loss of the ability to breathe spontaneously is insufficient for declaring death can be easily dispelled by consider-ing cases of neurological injury that deprive a patient of the ability to breathe and yet leave untouched the ability to engage in activities dependent on other parts of the CNS. Patients with high spinal cord injuries present such a condition: they remain awake and alert but dependent upon ventilators for respiratory support.

Furthermore, even the loss of *all* functions of the CNS is not a suf-ficient criterion for declaring death if this loss of function is not *irreversible*. Again, there are critical care cases that demonstrate the importance of this qualification—for instance, when a patient is in a deep, non-breathing ("apneic") coma during a critical emergency and the support of the ventilator allows time for CNS functions to return. In some cases like this, a full recovery of CNS functions oc-curs. More often, though, the functions that return will only be enough to leave the patient in a "vegetative state" that, if it persists, will be labeled a PVS (a *persistent* vegetative state). PVS will be discussed more fully in Part V, but the point here is that the deep, non-breathing coma that the patient was in prior to "waking" into the vegetative state could not have been *death* since the loss of functions proved to be reversible.

This discussion should make it clear why the condition typically called "brain death" and referred to in this report as "total brain failure" is called "irreversible apneic coma"[*] by some commentators. "Apneic" and "coma" describe the critical functional losses and "irreversible" adds the necessary qualification to rule out transient losses of these functions.

In view of these complications, how can a clinician determine whether a patient has suffered total brain failure? This question concerns the tests that must be conducted to distinguish patients with this condition from other brain-injured individuals for whom recovery of (at least some) brain functions remains possible. The next part takes up this issue directly.

II. The Diagnosis of Total Brain Failure

The diagnostic criteria that a physician uses to determine whether a patient has suffered total brain failure begin with the obvious but important requirement that the patient be in a completely unresponsive coma.[†] This means that the eyes are closed and no response whatsoever is made to any verbal or painful stimuli.

---

[*] See Chapter Two, Table 1.

[†] The discussion of testing for total brain failure in this section is meant only as a "layman's summary." For a more complete description the reader should consult the clinical literature, in particular, American Academy of Neurology, Quality Standards Subcommittee, "Practice Parameters for Determining Brain Death in Adults (Summary Statement)," *Neurology* 45, no. 5 (1995): 1012-4; and E. F. Wijdicks, "The Diagnosis of Brain Death," *N Engl J Med* 344, no. 16 (2001): 1215-21.

Another requirement for the diagnosis of total brain failure concerns the patient's history. The cause of the patient's brain injury cannot be hypothermia, poisoning, drug intoxication, or any such cause that brings about metabolic changes that can mimic the effects of total brain failure. The reason that a total brain failure diagnosis is ruled out in these cases is plain: A condition like this is often transient—it may clear up when the cause of the metabolic change passes out of the patient's system or is otherwise removed.*

If the patient being diagnosed is determined to be in a deep, unresponsive coma and none of the excluding causes just mentioned is present, then a battery of further tests must be conducted. These tests can be divided into two complementary groups: *clinical or bedside* tests and *laboratory or imaging* tests. The bedside tests are performed by trained clinicians, usually neurologists, and do not involve any high-tech instruments. The laboratory tests do involve such equipment and are intended to provide a more complete picture of what the clinician observes during the clinical examination.

With the clinical bedside tests for total brain failure, the clinician examines the comatose patient for any signs of *brainstem* function (See Figure 4). The functional status of this part of the brain is important for several reasons. First, the functions that depend on the brainstem are central to the basic work of the organism as a whole. This has already been noted with respect to the brainstem's (particularly, the medulla's) involvement in breathing. Brainstem function is also critical to an organism's conscious life. One part of the brainstem, known as the "reticular activating system," is essential for maintaining a state of wakefulness, which is a prerequisite for any of the activities associated with consciousness.

In addition to its significance for the patient's functional capacities, the condition of the brainstem also has a general diagnostic signifi-

---

* For a clinical case study of a patient who showed all the signs of total brain failure after a snake bite but then recovered after receiving an antidote, see R. Agarwal, N. Singh, and D. Gupta, "Is the Patient Brain-Dead?" *Emerg Med J* 23, no. 1 (2006): e5.

cance in most cases, for the brainstem is the most resilient part of the brain as a whole. As will be elaborated in Part III, if a brain injury has progressed to the point at which the brainstem retains no function, it has probably ravaged the more fragile parts of the brain as well. Thus, the bedside tests for brainstem function are tests for the extent of destruction both to the brainstem and to the parts of the brain "above the brainstem"—the so-called "higher centers."[*]

How, then, do the clinical tests determine the status of the brainstem? One marker of brainstem function has already been explored in depth: the signal that is sent from the respiratory centers to the muscles of respiration. Thus, the patient's *drive to breathe* must be tested with an apnea test. "Apnea" is the technical term for an inability to breathe. Although all patients who receive ventilator support need the machine's help to breathe, most are not so injured that they have no drive to breathe whatsoever. The purpose of the apnea test for total brain failure is to establish that the patient has *no* drive to bring air into the body even when the sensors in the brainstem are receiving an unambiguous signal that breathing is required.

Recall from the previous discussion that these sensors serve to trigger movement of the muscles of respiration when high levels of carbon dioxide in the blood are detected. In the apnea test, then, the ventilator is removed and the level of carbon dioxide in the patient's bloodstream is permitted to increase beyond the point that

---

[*] The exception to the rule discussed in the text is a case where a primary lesion of the brainstem leads to the diagnostic signs that usually indicate total brain failure. In such a case, the condition of the brainstem is not itself a reliable indicator of the condition of the higher centers of the brain. Among those who accept the neurological standard for determining death, there is controversy about the vital status of the patient about whom *all that is known* is the condition of the brainstem. See S. Laureys, "Science and Society: Death, Unconsciousness and the Brain," *Nat Rev Neurosci* 6, no. 11 (2005): 901-02; J. L. Bernat, "On Irreversibility as a Prerequisite for Brain Death Determination," *Adv Exp Med Biol* 550 (2004): 166; and C. Pallis and D. H. Harley, *ABC of Brainstem Death*, Second ed. (London: BMJ Publishing Group, 1996): 11-12. For the purposes of this report, such patients are excluded from the group considered to have "total brain failure."

would normally trigger inhalation.* If the examining clinicians see any signs that the chest is moving, the brainstem clearly has some vitality left and thus the patient cannot be diagnosed with total brain failure.

Another set of indicators of brainstem function are the automatic responses or "brainstem reflexes." Elicited by appropriate stimuli, these include the gag reflex, the cough reflex, and the reflex to move the eyes in certain ways under certain conditions (e.g., when the head is moved, which normally causes the oculocephalic reflex or doll's eyes phenomenon, or when cold water is injected into the ear canal). The examining clinicians will provide the appropriate stimuli to detect the presence or absence of these reflexes. If any are present, a diagnosis of total brain failure is ruled out.

In summary, a diagnosis of total brain failure can be made only when each of the following four conditions has been met:

1. The patient has a documented history of injury that does not suggest a potentially transient cause of symptoms, such as hypothermia or drug intoxication.

2. The patient is verified to be in a completely unresponsive coma.

3. The patient demonstrates no brainstem reflexes.

---

* The patient is prepared for this test by receiving, in advance, an elevated level of circulating oxygen that will prevent any further damage to tissues while the test is being carried out. Some inconsistencies in the way the apnea test is carried out in different places—including whether it is required at all in some countries—have been documented. For more information, see E. F. Wijdicks, "Brain Death Worldwide: Accepted Fact but No Global Consensus in Diagnostic Criteria," *Neurology* 58, no. 1 (2002): 20-5; R. Vardis and M. M. Pollack, "Increased Apnea Threshold in a Pediatric Patient with Suspected Brain Death," *Crit Care Med* 26, no. 11 (1998): 1917-9; and R. J. Brilli and D. Bigos, "Apnea Threshold and Pediatric Brain Death," *Crit Care Med* 28, no. 4 (2000): 1257.

4. The patient shows no drive to breathe during the apnea test.

A result indicating that all of these conditions have been met must be confirmed with a second examination some hours after the initial positive results are obtained. The appropriate length of time between these examinations is a matter of some debate. According to a consensus statement developed by the American Academy of Neurology in 1995, "[A] repeat clinical evaluation [six] hours later is recommended, but this interval is arbitrary."[1] The six-hour interval is far shorter than the interval recommended by the medical consultants to the President's Commission in 1981: they suggested twelve hours in cases of a non-anoxic etiology (e.g., head trauma of any kind, a stroke) and twenty-four hours in cases of an anoxic origin (e.g., a heart attack that leads to temporary cessation of circulation to the brain).[2] The standard interval between examinations also varies from one country to another, ranging from two hours to twenty-four hours.[3]

Questions about the appropriate interval between examinations are related to questions about what laboratory or imaging tests are needed to confirm the clinical diagnosis. These tests include the electroencephalogram (EEG), tests for evoked responses (brainstem auditory evoked potentials, somatic evoked potentials, and motor evoked responses), and tests for blood flow through the vessels that feed the brain (classic arteriography, radioisotope studies, and transcranial Doppler ultrasonography).[4] Standard practice in the United States dictates that these tests should be optional, to be used by the clinician in difficult cases—for example, when some factor interferes with clinical testing or when there is a need to abbreviate the interval before a second round of testing. In some other countries, the laboratory tests are mandatory.[5]

Neurologist James Bernat, a noted expert on the brain and its injuries, has recommended that tests of intracranial blood flow be included among the routine tests for total brain failure (or "brain death") in the United States.[6] These imaging tests are particularly useful for determining whether the pathophysiological events that lead to total brain failure have in fact occurred. Those events will be described and clarified in Part III.

First, however, we should make note of some well-known obstacles to making the diagnosis of total brain failure in infants and children. These obstacles have led to recommendations for longer observation times between clinical examinations, more extensive use of imaging tests, and modifications to the tests themselves.[7]

For both children and adults, some studies have shown that testing for the condition known as "brain death" is not always carried out in a consistent way from one institution to another.[8] In light of the very serious consequences of this diagnosis, it is especially important to ensure that variations in practice do not lead to errors or abuse.

III. Total Brain Failure: Pathophysiology

The question addressed in Part II was, How can the clinician distinguish the patient with total brain failure from other brain-injured patients? In this part we turn to the question, What events in the brain and body of the patient lead to total brain failure? As we have indicated, a diagnosis of total brain failure involves a judgment that the brainstem and the structures above it have been destroyed and therefore have lost the capacity to function ever again. In most cases, however, this destruction did not accompany the initial injury to the brain but instead came about through a self-perpetuating cascade of events—events that progressively damaged more and more tissue and finally destroyed the brainstem.

The source of this self-perpetuating cascade of damaging events is the rigidity of the skull, which, after injury, can cause elevated pressure in the cranial vault that holds and usually protects the brain. Consider the three most common injuries leading to total brain failure. These are (1) head trauma (sustained, for example, in an automobile accident or as a result of a gunshot wound), (2) cerebrovascular accident (i.e., "stroke"), and (3) cerebral anoxia (deprivation of oxygen) secondary to cardiac arrest. These three different causes have a common effect: severe damage to the cells comprising the tissues of the brain, that is, to the neurons and the cellular networks that they form. This damage leads, in turn, to edema, the abnormal accumulation of fluid. With little or no space in which to expand, the swelling brain suffers steady increases in intracranial pressure (ICP). Elevated ICP prevents oxygen-laden blood from making its way up and into the cranial cavity and thus deprives brain tissues of essential nutrients. This, in turn, leads to additional damage, which leads to more edema and swelling. Neurologist Alan Shewmon describes the result:

> A vicious cycle is established in which decreasing cerebral perfusion and increasing cerebral edema reinforce one another until blood no longer enters the cranial cavity and the brain herniates though the tentorium and foramen magnum.[9]

The herniation that Shewmon refers to here can crush the brainstem, leading to the functional losses that are revealed by the examination for total brain failure. That condition is the end point of a vicious cycle—the point at which the brain, including its lower centers in the brainstem, has been rendered permanently dysfunctional.

This description of the physiological events that lead to total brain failure shows the utility of yet another term for the clinical state under discussion: "total brain infarction."* An "infarction" is defined as a "sudden insufficiency of arterial or venous blood supply...that produces a macroscopic area of necrosis."[10] When death is declared based on the currently accepted neurological standard, the self-perpetuating cascade of events in the brain following the initial injury has run its full course. "Running its full course," in this context, means that total destruction of the brain has occurred due to infarction or lack of blood supply—hence, "total brain infarction."

---

* See Chapter Two, Table 1.

Bedside tests that establish loss of all brainstem reflexes can show that the destructive storm has indeed run its course, because the brainstem is often the last structure to be compromised in this process. Confirmatory tests and, in particular, various sorts of angiography (measurements of cranial blood flow) can be very useful in confirming that the gross infarction that is required for a diagnosis of total brain failure has actually occurred.[11]

At this point, it is important to take note of some qualifications regarding the word "total" in the context of total brain failure. One medically based objection to the neurological standard for determining death is based on a particular understanding of this word. Critics point out that the destructive storm that leads to "total" brain failure can leave certain areas of the brain intact. Again, from the description provided by Shewmon:

It should be mentioned that the self-destruction of the brain is not complete. Islands of sick but not totally necrosed brain tissue sometimes remain, presumably due to inhomogeneities of intracranial pressure and/or blood supply from extracranial collateral vessels.[12]

When the preserved areas of the brain do not support any recognizable function, this lack of total anatomical annihilation is less troubling. As the President's Commission noted in its report, the neurological standard for death requires an irreversible loss of all brain functions, not complete anatomical destruction of the tissue.[13] Isolated metabolic or electrical activity in dispersed cells cannot be a sign that a patient is still alive; after all, such activity, supporting no function of the whole organism, can continue even in some cells of a corpse after the heart has stopped beating.

As critics have pointed out, however, the physiological facts are not so simple.[14] In some cases, the preserved tissue in a body with total brain failure actually does support certain isolated functions of the brain. Most notably, some patients with total brain failure do not exhibit the condition known as "diabetes insipidus." This condition develops when a hormone known as ADH (anti-diuretic hormone) is not released by a part of the brain known as "the posterior pituitary." The absence of diabetes insipidus suggests that the "dead" brain is continuing to secrete the hormone; thus, at least with regard to this one function, the brain remains functional. It is therefore a fair criticism of the neurological standard, as enshrined in the UDDA, that "all functions of the entire brain, including the brain-stem" are not, in fact, always irreversibly lost when the diagnosis is made.[*]

It may be helpful to emphasize that the word "total" in the phrase,"total brain failure," refers to the fact that the brain injury has reached the *endpoint* of a process of self-perpetuating destruction of neural tissue. In any event, whether or not the word "total" is justified, the patient diagnosed with total brain failure is in a condition of profound incapacity, diagnostically distinct from all other cases of severe injury. Whether this state of profound incapacity warrants a determination of death remains a matter of debate, with advocates of the neurological standard arguing that it does, while critics maintain that it does not. The release of ADH and other signs of isolated brain function do not settle the fundamental issue: *Is the organism as a whole still present?*

IV. Total Brain Failure: "Health" and "Prognosis"

Contemporary controversies about total brain failure as a suitable standard for human death focus attention on certain medical findings and on conclusions drawn from these findings by critics of today's practice. In this part, we will examine two important types of such findings which are often cited as highly relevant to the debate.

---

[*] Researchers suspect that function in the posterior pituitary is preserved partly because its (extradural) arterial source is distinct from that which feeds other tissue of the brain. The damage that is due to the rise in intracranial pressure, which leads to total brain failure, can spare these extradural arteries so that a portion of pituitary is preserved. For discussion of this point, see E. F. Wijdicks and J. L. Atkinson, "Pathophysiologic Responses to Brain Death," in *Brain Death*, ed. E. F. Wijdicks (Philadelphia: Lippincott Williams & Wilkins, 2001).

A. "Somatic Health"

The first type of medical finding concerns the "somatic health" of the body of a patient diagnosed with total brain failure (or "whole brain death"). The appropriateness of the word "health" in this context is, itself, a point of contention. If the body is a cadaver then, of course, it is no longer fitting to speak about its "health." Nonetheless, *something like health* is still present in the body of a patient with this diagnosis. This can be seen clearly in the "donor management" procedures that are a regular part of organ retrieval from heart-beating ("brain dead") cadavers. These procedures aim to maintain the body in a relatively stable state of homeostasis so that the patient's heart does not stop beating prior to surgery and the organs procured remain as healthy as possible.[15] Thus, there is some degree of somatically integrated activity that persists in the bodies of patients who have been declared dead according to the neurological standard. The bodies of these patients do not "come apart" immediately upon succumbing to total brain failure.

This point deserves emphasis because of the history of the debate about the neurological standard for death in the United States. In that debate, certain exaggerated claims have been made about the "loss of somatic integration" that occurs in a body with a destroyed brain. A good example of this can be found in a very influential paper published in 1981 by James Bernat, Charles Culver, and Bernard Gert. In that paper, they assert the following:

> This criterion [whole brain death] is perfectly correlated with the permanent cessation of functioning of the organism as a whole because the brain is necessary for the functioning of the organism as a whole. It integrates, generates, interrelates, and controls complex bodily activities. A patient on a ventilator with a totally destroyed brain is merely a group of artificially maintained subsystems since the organism as a whole has ceased to function.[16]

The claim that the body of a patient diagnosed with "whole brain death" is a mere "group of artificially maintained subsystems" was repeated often enough to become established in the United States as the standard rationale for equating total brain failure with human death: patients with this condition are dead because the systems of the body do not work together *in an integrated way*.

But this standard rationale was soundly criticized in another influential paper, published by UCLA neurologist Alan Shewmon in 2001. In "The Brain and Somatic Integration: Insights Into the Standard Rationale for Equating 'Brain Death' With Death," Shewmon argues forcefully that patients who are positively and reliably diagnosed with "brain death" (total brain failure) continue to exhibit *many* functions that one can hardly avoid calling "somatically integrative." Examples include the maintenance of some degree of hemodynamic stability and body temperature, the elimination of wastes, the immune response to infection, the exhibiting of a stress response to the incision made for organ retrieval, and others.[17]

The reason that these somatically integrative activities continue, Shewmon rightly notes, is that the brain is not the *integrator* of the body's many and varied functions. In normal circumstances, the brainstem does play an important and complex role in supporting bodily integration. But no single structure in the body plays the role of an indispensable integrator. Integration, rather, is an emergent property of the whole organism—a property that does not depend upon directions from any one part, but is the product of the orchestration of multiple parts.

Based on his critique of the "somatic integration rationale," Shewmon draws the conclusion that there is no defensible biological account to justify the equation of total brain failure with human death. As he puts it, "If [brain death] is to be equated with death, therefore, it must be on the basis of an essentially *non-somatic, non-biological* concept of death."[18] In Chapter Four, we will re-examine the medical facts noted here to determine whether Shewmon's conclusion, repeated often by others, is warranted.

B. *"Prognosis"*

Just as it is paradoxical to talk about the "health" of the body of a patient who has been declared dead based on the neurological standard, it is also paradoxical to talk about the "prognosis" of that individual. Only a living creature can have a "prognosis," strictly speaking. Because our concern here is with the question of whether the patient with total brain failure is dead or alive, we should avoid language that implies that the matter is settled.

Hence, "prognosis," here, should be taken to have a very particular meaning—it refers to the likely timing of events that will result in the total collapse of the body's systems despite aggressive treatment to prevent that collapse. The President's Commission addressed "prognosis" in this sense when it claimed:

> In adults who have experienced irreversible cessation of the functions of the entire brain, this mechanically generated functioning can continue only a limited time because the heart usually stops beating within two to ten days. (An infant or small child who has lost all brain functions will typically suffer cardiac arrest within several weeks, although respiration and heartbeat can sometimes be maintained even longer).[19]

Most neurologists agree with this assessment of how long the body of a patient with total brain failure can persist even with aggressive treatment. Many have even based their confidence in the suitability of the neurological standard on the "fact" that bodies found to have no brainstem function will quickly become asystolic (i.e., have no heartbeat) no matter what help is given to them. The loss of all functions of the brain is typically referred to as a "point of no return," meaning no amount of medical effort can prevent the body from losing its integrity as an entropy-resistant system.[20]

As skeptics of today's neurological standard point out, there are two problems with this assessment. First, improvements in intensive care techniques over the years—prompted in part by the need for better "donor management" to procure usable organs—have made predictions of maximum survival time for bodies with total brain failure uncertain. Second, in practice, there turn out to be very few situations in which the truth of this matter can be tested. A diagnosis of total brain failure, when leading to a pronouncement of death, is a self-fulfilling prophesy: The patient with that diagnosis will become an organ donor (and the heart will stop in the process), or the ventilator will be withdrawn because it is understood to be "ventilating a corpse." As the late neurologist Ronald Cranford put it:

> It is impossible to know with certainty the extent of prolonged survival in brain death because a systematic clinical study in which the cardiac and circulatory functions are sustained for prolonged periods (weeks, months, or years) in a large number of patients is morally indefensible, extraordinarily expensive in terms of money and resources or manpower and intensive care unit beds, and legally prohibitive.[21]

For this reason, there is no effective way to determine how many patients could be stabilized in the condition of total brain failure and for how long. Uncontrolled observations must suffice. Such observations have been made in cases of patients who were pregnant at the time of their diagnosis with total brain failure. In some of these cases, efforts have been made to keep the body going until the fetus reaches viability. Eleven such cases are reported in a 2003 survey by Powner and Bernstein. According to these authors, no descriptions of unsuccessful attempts at fetal support after maternal brain death were found. The length of time that support continued after "brain death" ranged from thirty-six hours to 107 days.[22] These cases justify caution and skepticism toward sweeping claims about the total instability of the "brain dead" body and the imminent collapse of the body's systems.

V. Total Brain Failure and the Vegetative State

We conclude this chapter with an attempt to bring some clarity to a common misunderstanding of the difference between "whole brain death" and the condition known as the "vegetative state." Such confusion is exacerbated by the common and imprecise use of the term "brain dead" to describe patients who have *clearly not* been diagnosed with total brain failure and who do not exhibit the same level of incapacitation. Individuals such as Karen Ann Quinlan, Nancy Cruzan, and Terri Schiavo have been the subject of legal disputes and media attention because of family requests to withdraw various forms of life-sustaining treatment. With some frequency, these women have been inaccurately referred to as being "brain dead," when in fact they were all in a *persistent vegetative state* (PVS).

The initial clinical state of a patient who is eventually diagnosed with PVS may be similar to that of a patient diagnosed with total brain failure. But the previously described tests for total brain failure will provide the evidence to discriminate between the two groups: only the patient with total brain failure will show evidence of a completely destroyed brainstem. In the patient with a lesser brain injury, the brainstem, and possibly parts of the brain above the brainstem, will be found to be functionally preserved.

Although he or she might initially be in the same eyes-closed, unresponsive coma as the patient with total brain failure, the less injured patient will eventually emerge from this coma and display the typical signs of the vegetative state. These include opening the eyes, going through sleep/wake cycles, moving the limbs, breathing spontaneously, and, in some cases, displaying a minimal responsiveness to pain stimuli. Because spontaneous breathing, under the regulation of the medulla oblongata in the brainstem, resumes, the PVS patient will not need the continual support of the ventilator. In most cases, however, he or she will need to receive nourishment through a feeding tube. If such sustaining treatment and diligent nursing care are provided, a patient can survive for many years in a vegetative state.

Because it will be important to the discussion in Chapter Four, the question of "consciousness" in the PVS patient should be briefly addressed here. The degree of consciousness present in a patient in a vegetative state is a matter of some dispute. It is often said that PVS patients retain the capacity for wakefulness but have lost the capacity to be aware. This latter assertion, however, is increasingly controversial in light of recent findings indicating that at least some patients in a vegetative state retain a residual capacity for willful and consciously aware interaction with their surrounding environment.[23]

The cautionary advice of Steven Laureys, an expert on PVS and other brain-injured states, should be kept in mind:

> There is an irreducible philosophical limitation in knowing for certain whether any other being possesses a conscious life. Consciousness is a multifaceted subjective first-person experience and clinical evaluation is limited to evaluating patients' responsiveness to the environment. As previously discussed, patients in a vegetative state, unlike patients with brain death, can move extensively, and clinical studies have shown how difficult it is to differentiate 'automatic' from 'willed' movements. This results in an underestimation of behavioural signs of consciousness and, therefore, a misdiagnosis, which is estimated to occur in about one third of patients in a chronic vegetative state... Clinical testing for absence of consciousness is much more problematic than testing for absence of wakefulness, brainstem reflexes and apnoea in whole brain or brainstem death.[24]

Deciding whether ambiguous signs of wakeful life indicate consciousness is beyond the power of medicine, at least at this time, and possibly in principle. Thus, in cases where wakefulness is evident (as it is for PVS patients), there is good reason to be very cautious about assuming that conscious life is extinguished.

VI. Total Brain Failure: From Clinical Presentation and Pathophysiology to the Philosophical Debate

In this chapter, we have sought to explicate and clarify the condition usually called "brain death" or "whole brain death," emphasizing developments in medical understanding since the President's Commission published its seminal work in 1981. In certain respects, the medical facts have introduced complications for those who would defend the equation of this condition with the death of the human being: Patients diagnosed with total brain failure may retain certain limited brain functions (such as the secretion of ADH to regulate urine output), and they certainly retain enough somatic integrity to challenge claims that the body immediately becomes "a disorganized collection of organs" once the brainstem is disabled. In addition, advances in intensive care techniques, displayed in cases of prolonged somatic "survival" after "whole brain death," challenge claims that the body cannot continue in its artificially supported state beyond a short window of time.

Alongside these challenging findings, however, are facts that confirm the diagnostic and pathophysiological distinctiveness of total brain failure. Patients with this degree of injury are, indeed, singled out by the battery of tests (bedside and laboratory) first outlined and recommended by the Harvard committee in 1968. Moreover, no patient diagnosed with "total brain failure" has ever recovered the capacity to breathe spontaneously or shown *any* sign of consciousness—including the minimal and ambiguous signs routinely displayed by patients who emerge into the vegetative state.

Having drawn this detailed picture of the medical facts, we can now address the fundamental philosophical question of this report, *Are patients diagnosed with total brain failure (or "whole brain death"), by virtue of this fact, truly dead?*

ENDNOTES

[1] American Academy of Neurology, Quality Standards Subcommittee, "Practice Parameters for Determining Brain Death in Adults (Summary Statement)," *Neurology* 45, no. 5 (1995): 1014.

[2] President's Commission for the Study of Ethical Problems in Medicine and Biomedical and Behavioral Research, Report of the Medical Consultants on the Diagnosis of Death, "Guidelines for the Determination of Death," *JAMA* 246, no. 19 (1981): 2184-6.

[3] E. F. Wijdicks, "Brain Death Worldwide: Accepted Fact but No Global Consensus in Diagnostic Criteria," *Neurology* 58, no. 1 (2002): 20-5.

[4] See F. Plum, "Clinical Standards and Technological Confirmatory Tests in Diagnosing Brain Death," in *The Definition of Death: Contemporary Controversies*, ed. S. J. Youngner, R. M. Arnold, and R. Schapiro (Baltimore: The Johns Hopkins University Press, 1999) 34-65; and E. F Wijdicks, "The Diagnosis of Brain Death," *N Engl J Med* 344, no. 16 (2001): 1215-21.

[5] Wijdicks, "Brain Death Worldwide," 20-5.

[6] J. L. Bernat, "On Irreversibility as a Prerequisite for Brain Death Determination," *Adv Exp Med Biol* 550 (2004): 161-7; and J. L. Bernat, "The Whole-Brain Concept of Death Remains Optimum Public Policy," *J Law Med Ethics* 34, no. 1 (2006): 40.

[7] See Report of the Medical Consultants on the Diagnosis of Death, "Guidelines for the Determination of Death," 2184-6; Task Force for the Determination of Brain Death in Children, "Guidelines for the Determination of Brain Death in Children," *Neurology* 37, no. 6 (1987): 1077-8; R. Vardis and M. M. Pollack, "Increased Apnea Threshold in a Pediatric Patient with Suspected Brain Death, " *Crit Care Med* 26, no. 11 (1998): 1917-9; R. J. Brilli and D. Bigos, "Apnea Threshold and Pediatric Brain Death," *Crit Care Med* 28, no. 4 (2000): 1257; S. Ashwal, "Clinical Diagnosis and Confirmatory Testing of Brain Death in Children," in *Brain Death*, ed. E. F. Wijdicks (Philadelphia: Lippincott Williams & Wilkins, 2001); and K. J. Banasiak and G. Lister, "Brain Death in Children," *Curr Opin Pediatr* 15, no. 3 (2003): 288-93.

[8] See R. E. Mejia and M. M. Pollack, "Variability in Brain Death Determination Practices in Children," *JAMA* 274, no. 7 (1995): 550-3; M. Y. Wang, P. Wallace, and J. P. Gruen, "Brain Death Documentation: Analysis and Issues," *Neurosurgery* 51, no. 3 (2002): 731-6; M. Y. Chang, L. A. McBride, and M. A. Ferguson, "Variability in Brain Death Declaration Practices in Pediatric Head Trauma Patients," *Pediatr Neurosurg* 39, no. 1 (2003): 7-9; and D. J. Powner, M. Hernandez, and T. E. Rives, "Variability Among Hospital Policies for Determining Brain Death in Adults," *Crit Care Med* 32, no. 6 (2004): 1284-8.

[9] D. A. Shewmon, "Recovery from 'Brain Death': A Neurologist's Apologia," *Linacre Q* 64, no. 1 (1997): 30-96.

[10] T. L. Stedman, *Stedman's Medical Dictionary*, 26th ed. (Baltimore: Lippincott Williams & Wilkins, 1995): 868.

[11] Bernat, "Irreversibility as a Prerequisite," 161-7.

[12] Shewmon, "Neurologist's Apologia," 40.

[13] *Defining Death*, 75-76.

[14] See, for instance, A. Halevy and B. Brody, "Brain Death: Reconciling Definitions, Criteria, and Tests," *Ann Intern Med* 119, no. 6 (1993): 519-25.

[15] A discussion of the physiological consequences of total brain failure from the perspective of donor management is provided in R. Arbour, "Clinical Management of the Organ Donor," *AACN Clin Issues* 16, no. 4 (2005): 551-80. Also see J. M. Darby et al., "Approach to Management of the Heartbeating 'Brain Dead' Organ Donor," *JAMA* 261, no. 15 (1989): 2222-8; and D. Wikler and A. J. Weisbard, "Appropriate Confusion over 'Brain Death'," *JAMA* 261, no. 15 (1989): 2246.

[16] J. L. Bernat, C. M. Culver, and B. Gert, "On the Definition and Criterion of Death," *Ann Intern Med* 94, no. 3 (1981): 391.

[17] A. D. Shewmon, "The Brain and Somatic Integration: Insights into the Standard Biological Rationale for Equating 'Brain Death' With Death," *J Med Philos* 26, no. 5 (2001): 457-78. For a more complete list of integrated functions that persist after "brain death," see Chapter Four, Table 2.

[18] Ibid., 473.

[19] *Defining Death*, 17.

[20] J. Korein, "The Problem of Brain Death: Development and History," *Ann NY Acad Sci* 315 (1978): 19-38.

[21] R. Cranford, "Even the Dead Are Not Terminally Ill Anymore," *Neurology* 51, no. 6 (1998): 1531.

[22] D. J. Powner and I. M. Bernstein, "Extended Somatic Support for Pregnant Women after Brain Death," *Crit Care Med* 31, no. 4 (2003): 1241-9. This survey includes sources for both pregnancy cases and non-pregnancy cases of prolonged survival after a diagnosis of "brain death."

[23] A. M. Owen et al., "Detecting Awareness in the Vegetative State," *Science* 313, no. 5792 (2006): 1402; and A. M. Owen et al., "Using Functional Magnetic Resonance Imaging to Detect Covert Awareness in the Vegetative State," *Arch Neurol* 64, no. 8 (2007): 1098-1102.

[24] S. Laureys, "Death, Unconsciousness and the Brain," *Nat Rev Neurosci* 6, no. 11 (2005): 904-05. Citations omitted.

CHAPTER FOUR

THE PHILOSOPHICAL DEBATE

Why do we describe the central question of this inquiry as a *philosophical* question? We do so, in part, because this question cannot be settled by appealing exclusively to clinical or pathophysiological facts. Those facts were our focus in the previous chapters in which we sought to clarify important features of "total brain failure," a condition diagnosed in a well-defined subset of comatose, ventilator-dependent patients. As a condition, it is the terminus of a course of pathophysiological events, the effects of which account for certain clinically observable signs (all manifestations of an incapacitated brainstem) and for confirmatory results obtained through selected imaging tests. A patient diagnosed with this condition will never recover brain-dependent functions, including the capacity to breathe and the capacity to exhibit even minimal signs of conscious life. If the patient is sustained with life-supporting technologies, this condition need not lead immediately to somatic disintegration or failure of other organ systems. These facts are all crucial to answering the question, *Is a human being with total brain failure dead?* But determining the significance of these facts presents challenges for philosophical analysis and interpretation.

In this chapter, we set forth and explore two positions on this philosophical question. One position rejects the widely accepted consensus that the current neurological standard is an ethically valid one for determining death. The other position defends the consensus, taking the challenges posed in recent years as opportunities to strengthen the philosophical rationale for the neurological standard.

At the outset, it is important to note what is common to these two opposing positions. *First, both reject the idea that death should be treated*

49

merely as a legal construct or as a matter of social agreement. Instead, both embrace the idea that a standard for determining death must be defensible on biological as well as philosophical grounds. That is to say, both positions respect the *biological reality* of death. At some point, after all, certainty that a body is no longer a living whole *is* attainable. The impressive technological advances of the last several decades have done nothing to alter the reality of death, even if they have complicated the task of judging whether and when death has occurred in particular circumstances. In light of such complications, however, both positions share the conclusion that a human being who is not known to be dead should be considered alive.

Second, neither position advocates loosening the standards for determining death on the basis of currently known clinical and pathophysiological facts. There is a well-developed third philosophical position that is often considered alongside the two that are the main focus of this chapter. This third position maintains that there can be two deaths—the death of the *person,* a being distinguished by the capacities for thought, reason, and feeling, and the death of the *body* or the *organism.* From the perspective of this third philosophical position, an individual who suffers a brain injury that leaves him incapacitated with regard to certain specifically human powers is rightly regarded as "dead as a person." The still living body that remains after this death is not a human being in the full sense. Philosopher John Lizza discusses the living organism left behind after the "person" has died in the following way:

> Advocates of a consciousness-related formulation of death do not consider such a being to be a living person. In their view, a person cannot persist through the loss of all brain function or even the loss of just those brain functions required for consciousness and other mental functions... [W]hat remains alive must be a different sort of being...a form of life created by medical technology... Whereas a person is normally transformed into a corpse at his or her death, technology has intervened in this natural process and has made it possible...for a person's remains to take the form of an artificially sustained, living organism devoid

of the capacity for consciousness and any other mental function.[1]

Thus, advocates of this third position effectively maintain that in certain cases there can be two deaths rather than one. In such cases, they argue, a body that has ceased to be a person (having "died" the first death) can be treated as deceased—at least in certain ways. For example, according to some advocates of this position, it would be permissible to remove the organs of such individuals while their hearts continue to beat. The patients most often cited as potential heart-beating organ donors, based on this concept of death, are PVS patients and anencephalic newborns (babies born with very little, if any, brain matter other than the brainstem). Organ retrieval in such cases might entail the administration of sedatives to the allegedly "person-less" patient because some signs of continued "biological life" (such as the open eyes and spontaneous breathing of the PVS patient) would be distracting and disturbing to the surgeons who procure the patient's organs.

Serious difficulties afflict the claim that something that can be called "death" has occurred even as the body remains alive. One such difficulty is that there is no way to know that the "specifically human powers" are irreversibly gone from a body that has suffered any injury shy of total brain failure. In Chapter Three, we cited neurologist Steven Laureys's observation that it is impossible to ascertain scientifically the inward state of an individual—and features of this inward state (e.g., thinking and feeling) are always cited as marks of a distinctively *human* or *personal* life. It is very important here to recall the marked differences in appearance between the individual with total brain failure and the individual with another "consciousness-compromising" condition. The latter displays several ambiguous signs—moving, waking up, and groaning, among others—while the former remains still and closed off from the world in clinically ascertainable ways.[2]

A related problem with this "two deaths" position is that it expands the concept of death beyond the core meaning it has had throughout human history. Human beings are members of the larger family of living beings, and it is a fundamental truth about living beings that every individual—be it plant or animal—eventually dies. Recent advances in technology offer no warrant for jettisoning the age-old idea that it is not as persons that we die, but rather as members of the family of living beings and as animals in particular. The terminus of the transformation that occurs when a human being is deprived by injury of certain mental capacities, heartbreaking as it is, is not *death*. We should note, again, that some technological interventions administered to the living might be deemed *futile*—that is, ineffective at reversing or ameliorating the course of disease or injury—and that an ethically valid decision might be made to withdraw or withhold such interventions. There is no need, however, to call an individual *already dead* in order to justify refraining from such futile interventions.

In summary, the two positions that we present in this chapter share the conviction that death is a single phenomenon marking the end of the life of a biological organism. Death is the definitive end of life and is something more complete and final than the mere loss of "personhood."

I. Position One: There Is No Sound Biological Justification for Today's Neurological Standard

The neurological standard for death based on total brain failure relies fundamentally on the idea that the phenomenon of death can be *hidden*. The metaphor employed by the President's Commission and cited in Chapter One expresses this idea: When a ventilator supports the body's vital functions, this technological intervention obscures our view of the phenomenon. What seem to be signs of continued life in an injured body are, in fact, misleading artifacts of the technological intervention and obstacles to ascertaining the truth. To consult brain-based functions, then, is to look through a "second window" in order to see the actual condition of the body.

The critical thrust of Position One can be summarized in this way: There is no reliable "second window" on the phenomenon of death. If its presence is not made known by the signs that have always accompanied it—by breathing lungs and a beating heart—then there is no way to state with confidence that death has occurred. Only when all would agree that the body is ready for burial can that body, with confidence, be described as dead. If blood is still circulating and nutrients and oxygen are still serving to power the work of diverse cells, tissues, and organ systems, then the body in which these processes are ongoing cannot be deemed a corpse.

Soon after the Harvard committee argued that patients who meet the criteria for "irreversible coma" are already dead, some philosophers and other observers of the committee's work advanced an opposing view. The counterarguments presented then by one such philosopher, Hans Jonas, are still useful in framing the objections raised today against the neurological standard. In his 1974 essay, "Against the Stream," Jonas dissented from the Harvard committee's equation of "irreversible coma" and death and counseled, instead, a conservative course of action:

> We do not know with certainty the borderline between life and death, and a definition cannot substitute for knowledge. Moreover, we have sufficient grounds for suspecting that the artificially supported condition of the comatose patient may still be one of life, however reduced—i.e., for doubting that, even with the brain function gone, he is completely dead. In this state of marginal ignorance and doubt the only course to take is to lean over backward toward the side of possible life.[3]

With these words, Jonas underscored a point that is pivotal to Position One: There can be uncertainty as to where the line between life and death falls even if we are certain that death is a biologically real event. In patients with total brain failure, the transition from living body to corpse is in some measure a mystery, one that may be beyond the powers of science and medicine to penetrate and determine with the finality that is possible when most human beings die.

Have advances in the scientific and clinical understanding of the spectrum of neurological injury shown that Jonas's stance of principled (and therefore cautious) uncertainty was incorrect? Today we have a more fine-grained set of categories of, as he put it, "artificially supported...comatose patients"—some of whom meet the criteria for total brain failure and others who have hope of recovering limited or full mental function. Only the first group is considered to be dead by today's "brain death" defenders. Even with respect to this group, however, there is still reason to wonder if our knowledge of their condition is adequate for labeling them as dead. If there are "sufficient grounds," as Jonas put it, for suspecting that their condition may still be one of life, then a stance of principled and hence cautious uncertainty is still the morally right one to take.

This line of inquiry brings us to Shewmon's criticisms, summarized earlier in Chapter Three, of the accepted pathophysiological and clinical picture of patients with "brain death" (total brain failure). Do Shewmon's criticisms constitute the "sufficient grounds" to which Jonas appeals? To answer this question, these criticisms and the evidence supporting them must first be considered in greater depth.

In 1998, the journal *Neurology* published an article by Shewmon entitled, "Chronic 'Brain Death': Meta-Analysis and Conceptual Consequences." In that article, Shewmon cites evidence for the claim that neither bodily disintegration nor cessation of heartbeat *necessarily* and *imminently* ensues after brain death.[4] Shewmon's evidence is drawn from more than one hundred documented cases that demonstrate survival past one week's time, with one case of survival for more than fourteen years.[*] Furthermore, he demonstrates that such factors as age, etiology, and underlying somatic integrity variably affect the survival probability of "brain dead" patients. Observing that asystole (the absence of cardiac contractions colloquially known as "flatline") does not necessarily follow from "brain death," Shewmon concludes that it is the overall integrity of the body (the

---

[*] This patient experienced a cardiac arrest in January 2004, more than twenty years after the diagnosis of "brain death." A report on the case, including the brain-only autopsy performed, appears in S. Repertinger, et al., "Long Survival Following Bacterial Meningitis-Associated Brain Destruction," *J Child Neurol* 21, no. 7 (2006): 591-5.

"underlying somatic plasticity") *rather than the condition of the brain* that exerts the strongest influence on survival. These facts seem to contradict the dominant view that the loss of brain function, in and of itself, leads the body to "fall apart" and eventually to cease circulating blood.

Critics of this meta-analysis have challenged the data on which Shewmon based his conclusions, claiming that many of the patients in the cases that he compiles might not have been properly diagnosed with whole brain death (in our usage, total brain failure). They also point out the rarity with which such cases are encountered, compared with the frequency of rapid descent to asystole for patients accurately diagnosed.[*] To point out the rarity of prolonged survival, however, is to admit that the phenomenon does, in some cases, occur. Whether it might occur more often is difficult to judge because patients with total brain failure are rarely treated with aggressive, life-sustaining interventions for an extended time.

If it is possible—albeit rare—for a body without a functioning brain to "hold itself together" for an indefinite period of time, then how can the condition of total brain failure be equated with biological death? Or, to put the question in Jonas's terms, does this fact not give "sufficient grounds" for suspecting that such patients might still be alive, although severely injured? The case for uncertainty about the line between life and death is further strengthened by considering the somatic processes that clearly continue in the body of a patient with total brain failure.

In a paper published in the *Journal of Medicine and Philosophy* in 2001, Shewmon details the integrated functions that continue in a body in the condition of "brain death." Table 2 reproduces a list of somatically integrative functions that are, in Shewmon's words, "*not*

---

[*] Wijdicks and Bernat, in a response to the Shewmon article, commented: "These cases are anecdotes yearning for a denominator." E. F. Wijdicks and J. L. Bernat, "Chronic 'Brain Death': Meta-Analysis and Conceptual Consequences," *Neurology* 53, no. 6 (1999): 1538-45.

mediated by the brain and possessed by at least some [brain dead] bodies."[5]

Table 2: Physiological Evidence of "Somatic Integration"[6]

- Homeostasis of a countless variety of mutually interacting chemicals, macromolecules and physiological parameters, through the functions especially of liver, kidneys, cardiovascular and endocrine systems, but also of other organs and tissues (e.g., intestines, bone and skin in calcium metabolism; cardiac atrial natriuretic factor affecting the renal secretion of renin, which regulates blood pressure by acting on vascular smooth muscle; etc.);
- Elimination, detoxification and recycling of cellular wastes throughout the body;
- Energy balance, involving interactions among liver, endocrine systems, muscle and fat;
- Maintenance of body temperature (albeit at a lower than normal level and with the help of blankets);
- Wound healing, capacity for which is diffuse throughout the body and which involves organism-level, teleological interaction among blood cells, capillary endothelium, soft tissues, bone marrow, vasoactive peptides, clotting and clot lysing factors (maintained by the liver, vascular endothelium and circulating leucocytes in a delicate balance of synthesis and degradation), etc.;
- Fighting of infections and foreign bodies through interactions among the immune system, lymphatics, bone marrow, and microvasculature;
- Development of a febrile response to infection;
- Cardiovascular and hormonal stress responses to unanesthetized incision for organ retrieval;
- Successful gestation of a fetus in a [brain dead] pregnant woman;
- Sexual maturation of a [brain dead] child;
- Proportional growth of a [brain dead] child.

Readers not well-versed in human physiology might find this list hard to follow. Its significance, however, can be simply stated: It enumerates many clearly identifiable and observable physiological mechanisms. These mechanisms account for the continued health of vital organs in the bodies of patients diagnosed with total brain failure and go a long way toward explaining the lengthy survival of such patients in rare cases. In such cases, globally coordinated work continues to be performed by multiple systems, all directed toward the sustained functioning of the body as a whole. If being alive as a biological organism requires being a whole that is more than the mere sum of its parts, then it would be difficult to deny that the body of a patient with total brain failure can still be alive, at least in some cases.

None of this contradicts the claim that total brain failure is a unique and profound kind of *incapacitation*—and one that may very well warrant or even morally *require* the withdrawal of life-sustaining interventions. According to some defenders of the concept of medical futility, there is no obligation to begin or to continue treatment when that treatment cannot achieve any good or when it inflicts disproportionate burdens on the patient who receives it or on his or her family. Writing many years before the somatic state and the prognostic possibilities of total brain failure were well-characterized, Jonas emphasized the need to accept that sustaining life and prolonging dying is not always in the patient's interest:

> The question [of interventions to sustain the patient] cannot be answered by decreeing that death has already occurred and the body is therefore in the domain of things; rather it is by holding, e.g., that it is humanly not justified—let alone demanded—to artificially prolong the life of a brainless body...the physician can, indeed should, turn off the respirator and let the "definition of death" take care of itself by what then inevitably happens.[7]

To summarize, Position One does *not* insist that medicine or science can know that all or even some patients with total brain failure are still living. Rather, Position One makes two assertions in light of what we now know about the clinical presentation and the pathophysiology of total brain failure. The first is that there are "sufficient grounds" for doubt as to whether the patient with this condition has died. The second is that in the face of such persistent uncertainty, the only ethically valid course is to consider and treat such a patient as a still living human being. Finally, such respectful consideration and treatment does not preclude the ethical withdrawal or withholding of life-sustaining interventions, based on the judgment that such interventions are futile.

II. Position Two: There *Is* a Sound Biological Justification for Today's Neurological Standard

Position One is the voice of "principled and hence cautious uncertainty." We should not claim to know facts about life and death that are beyond the limits of our powers to discern, especially when the consequence might be to place a human being beyond the essential and obligatory protections afforded to the living. The recent critical appraisals of total brain failure ("whole brain death") offered by Shewmon and others only underscore the limits to our ability to discern the line between life and death.

Position Two is also motivated by strong moral convictions about what is at stake in the debate: The bodies of deceased patients should not be ventilated and maintained as if they were still living human beings. The respect owed to the newly dead demands that such interventions be withdrawn. Their families should be spared unnecessary anguish over purported "options" for treatment. Maintaining the body for a short time to facilitate organ transplantation is a reasonable act of deference to the need for organs and to the opportunity for generosity on the part of the donor as well as the family. Notwithstanding this need and opportunity, the true moral challenge that faces us is to decide in each case whether the patient is living or has died. To help us meet that challenge, the clinical and pathophysiological facts that call the neurological standard into question should be re-examined and re-evaluated. On the basis of such a re-examination and re-evaluation, Position Two seeks to develop a better rationale for continuing to use the neurological standard to determine whether a human being has died.

A. *The Work of the Organism as a Whole*

Early defenders of the neurological standard of "whole brain death" relied on the plausible intuition that in order to be a living organism any animal, whether human or non-human, must be a *whole*. Ongoing biological activity in various cells or tissues is not in itself sufficient to mark the presence of a living organism. After all, some biological activity in cells and tissues remains for a time even in a body that all would agree is a corpse. Such activity signifies that disparate *parts* of the once-living organism remain, but not the organism *as a whole*. Therefore, if we try to specify the moment at which the "wholeness" of the body is lost, that moment must come before biological activity in all of its different cells or tissues has ceased. As Alexander Capron, former executive director of the President's Commission, has repeatedly emphasized, the fact that this moment is *chosen* does not mean that it is *arbitrary*; the choice is not arbitrary if it is made in accordance with the most reasonable interpretation of the biological facts that could be provided.[*]

The neurological standard's early defenders were not wrong to seek such a principle of wholeness. They may have been mistaken, however, in focusing on the *loss of somatic integration* as the critical sign that the organism is no longer a whole. They interpreted—plausibly but perhaps incorrectly— "an organism as a whole" to mean "an

---

[*]Capron comments: "In part, any definition 'is admittedly arbitrary in the sense of representing a choice,' as the President's Commission stated in defending the view that the brain's function is more central to human life than are other necessary organs... But the societally determined view of what constitutes death is not 'arbitrary in the sense of lacking reasons.' ...The 'cultural context' of the standards for determining death includes the generally held view that human death, like the death of any animal, is a natural event. Even in establishing their 'definition,' members of our society act on the basis that death is an event whose existence rests on certain criteria recognized rather than solely invented by human beings." A. M. Capron, "The Report of the President's Commission on the Uniform Determination of Death Act," in *Death: Beyond Whole Brain Criteria*, ed. R. Zaner (The Netherlands: Kluwer Academic Publishers, 1988), 156-57. See, also, A. M. Capron, "The Purpose of Death: A Reply to Professor Dworkin," *Indiana Law J* 48, no. 4 (1973): 640-6.

organism whose parts are working together in an integrated way." But, as we have seen, even in a patient with total brain failure, some of the body's parts continue to work together in an integrated way for some time—for example, to fight infection, heal wounds, and maintain temperature. If these kinds of integration were sufficient to identify the presence of a living "organism as a whole," total brain failure could not serve as a criterion for organismic death, and the neurological standard enshrined in law would not be philosophically well-grounded.

There may be, however, a more compelling account of *wholeness* that would support the intuition that after total brain failure the body is no longer an organismic whole and hence no longer alive. That account, which we develop here with Position Two, offers a superior defense of "total brain failure" as the standard for declaring death. With that account, death remains a condition of the organism as a whole and does not, therefore, merely signal the irreversible loss of so-called higher mental functions. But reliance on the concept of "integration" is abandoned and with it the false assumption that the brain is the "integrator" of vital functions. Determining whether an organism remains a *whole* depends on recognizing the persistence or cessation of the fundamental vital *work* of a living organism—the work of self-preservation, achieved through the organism's need-driven commerce with the surrounding world. When there is good reason to believe that an injury has irreversibly destroyed an organism's ability to perform its fundamental vital work, then the conclusion that the organism as a whole has died is warranted. Advocates of Position Two argue that this is the case for patients with total brain failure. To understand this argument, we must explore at some length this idea of an organism's "fundamental work."

All organisms have a *needy* mode of being. Unlike inanimate objects, which continue to exist through inertia and without effort, every organism persists only thanks to its own exertions. To preserve themselves, organisms *must*—and *can* and *do*—engage in commerce with the surrounding world. Their constant need for oxygenated air and nutrients is matched by their ability to satisfy that need, by engaging in certain activities, reaching out into the surrounding environment to secure the required sustenance. This is the definitive work of the organism *as an organism*. It is what an organism "does" and what distinguishes every organism from non-living things.* And it is what distinguishes a *living* organism from the dead body that it becomes when it dies.

The work of the organism, expressed in its commerce with the surrounding world, depends on three fundamental capacities:

1. Openness to the world, that is, receptivity to stimuli and signals from the surrounding environment.

2. The ability to act upon the world to obtain selectively what it needs.

3. The basic felt need that drives the organism to act as it must, to obtain what it needs and what its openness reveals to be available.

Appreciating these capacities as mutually supporting aspects of the organism's vital work will help us understand why an individual with total brain failure should be declared dead, even when ventilator-supported "breathing" masks the presence of death.

To preserve itself, an organism must be open to the world. Such openness is manifested in different ways and at many levels. In higher animals, including man, it is evident most obviously in consciousness or felt awareness, even in its very rudimentary forms. When a PVS patient tracks light with his or her eyes, recoils in response to pain, swallows liquid placed in the mouth, or goes to sleep and wakes up, such behaviors—although they may not indicate *self*-consciousness—testify to the organism's essential, vital openness to its surrounding world. An organism that behaves in such a way cannot be dead.

---

* The account here focuses on the details of organismic life that are manifested in the "higher animals" or, perhaps more precisely, the *mammals*. How these arguments might be modified and extended to other sorts of organisms (e.g., bacteria or plants) is beyond the scope of this discussion.

Self-preserving commerce with the world, however, involves more than just openness or receptivity. It also requires the ability to *act* on one's own behalf—to take in food and water and, even more basically, to breathe. Spontaneous breathing is an indispensable action of the higher animals that makes metabolism—and all other vital activity—possible. Experiencing a felt inner need to acquire oxygen (and to expel carbon dioxide) and perceiving the presence of oxygen in its environment, a living body is moved to act on the world (by contracting its diaphragm so that air will move into its lungs). An organism that breathes spontaneously cannot be dead.

Just as spontaneous breathing in itself reveals an organism's openness to and ability to act upon the world, it also reveals a third capacity critical to the organism's fundamental, self-preserving work: What animates the motor act of spontaneous breathing, in open commerce with the surrounding air, is the inner experience of need, manifesting itself as the drive to breathe. This need does not have to be consciously felt in order to be efficacious in driving respiration. It is clearly not consciously felt in a comatose patient who might be tested for a remaining rudimentary drive (e.g., with the "apnea" test). But even when the drive to breathe occurs in the absence of any self-awareness, its presence gives evidence of the organism's continued impulse to live. This drive is the organism's own impulse, exercised on its own behalf, and indispensable to its continued existence.[*]

---

[*] The significance of this account of breathing may be more apparent if we contrast it with the more reductive account provided by Shewmon in his influential 2001 paper that criticized a "somatic integration rationale" for a whole brain standard for human death. Shewmon wrote:

> If "breathing" is interpreted in the "bellows" sense—moving air in and out of the lungs—then it is indeed a brain-mediated function, grossly substituted in [brain dead] patients by a mechanical ventilator. But this is a function not only of the brain but also of the phrenic nerves, diaphragm and intercostal muscles; moreover, it is not a somatically integrative function or even a vitally necessary one... It is merely a condition for somatic integration itself. On the other hand, if "breathing" is understood in the sense of "respiration," which strictly

As a vital sign, the *spontaneous action of breathing* can and must be distinguished from the technologically supported, *passive condition of being ventilated* (i.e., of having one's "breathing" replaced by a mechanical ventilator). The natural work of breathing, even apart from consciousness or self-awareness, is itself a sure sign that the organism as a whole is doing the work that constitutes—and preserves—it as a whole. In contrast, artificial, non-spontaneous breathing produced by a machine is not such a sign. It does not signify an activity of the organism as a whole. It is not driven by *felt need*, and the exchange of gases that it effects is neither an achievement of the organism nor a sign of its genuine vitality. For this reason, it makes sense to say that the operation of the ventilator can obscure our view of the arrival of human death—that is, the death of the human organism as a working whole. A ventilator causes the patient's chest

---

speaking refers to the exchange of oxygen and carbon dioxide, then its locus is twofold: (1) across the alveolar lining of the lungs, and (2) at the biochemical level of the electron transport chain in the mitochondria of every cell in the body. (Shewmon, "Brain and Somatic Integration," 464.)

In his eagerness to debunk what he considers the myth of lost somatic integration, Shewmon fails to convey the essential character of breathing. We might summarize his account of breathing as follows:

Breathing = Inflation and deflation of a bellows + Diffusion at the alveoli + Cellular respiration

But Shewmon misses the critical element: the *drive* exhibited by the whole organism to bring in air, a drive that is fundamental to the constant, vital working of the whole organism. By ignoring the essentially *appetitive* nature of animal breathing, Shewmon's account misses the relevance of breathing as incontrovertible evidence that "the organism as a whole" continues to be *open to* and *at work upon* the world, achieving its own preservation. The breathing that keeps an organism alive is not merely the operation of a "bellows" for which a mechanical ventilator might substitute. Bringing air into the body is an integral part of an organism's mode of being as a *needy* thing. More air will be brought in if metabolic need demands it and the body *feels* that need, as for example during exercise or in a state of panic or injury. The "respiration" taking place at the cellular level can be understood adequately only in the context of the work of the whole organism—the work of breathing.

to heave and the lungs to fill and thereby *mimics* the authentic work of the organism. In fact, it mimics the work so well that it enables some systems of the body to keep functioning—but it does no more than that. The simulated "breathing" that the ventilator makes possible is not, therefore, a *vital sign:* It is not a sign that the organism is accomplishing its vital work and thus remains a living whole.[*]

We have examined the phenomenon of breathing in order to understand and explain a living organism's "needful openness" to the world—a needful openness lacking in patients with total brain failure. Having done this, however, we must also emphasize that an animal cannot be considered dead simply because it has lost the ability to breathe spontaneously. Even if the animal has lost that capacity, other vital capacities might still be present. For example, patients with spinal cord injuries may be permanently apneic or unable to breathe without ventilatory support and yet retain full or partial possession of their conscious faculties. Just as much as striving to breathe, signs of consciousness are incontrovertible evidence that a living organism, a patient, is alive.

If there are no signs of consciousness *and* if spontaneous breathing is absent *and* if the best clinical judgment is that these neurophysiological facts cannot be reversed, Position Two would lead us to conclude that a once-living patient has now died. Thus, on this account, total brain failure can continue to serve as a criterion for declaring death—not because it necessarily indicates complete loss of integrated somatic functioning, but because it is a sign that this

---

[*] If the view presented here is correct, that is, if the presence of spontaneous breathing truly reveals a persistent drive of the organism as a whole to live, we can better understand the force of a rhetorical question sometimes posed to those who view the loss of "higher" mental and psychological capacities as a sufficient criterion for declaring death. "Would you," they may be asked, "bury a patient who continues to breathe spontaneously?" Quite naturally, we recoil from such a thought, and we do so for reasons that the account given above makes clear. The striving of an animal to live, a striving that we can discern even in its least voluntary form (i.e., breathing), indicates that we still have among us a living being—and not a candidate for burial.

organism can no longer engage in the essential work that defines living things.

B. Comparison with the UK Standard

Although the terms may be different, the concepts presented here to defend the use of total brain failure as a reasonable standard for death are not wholly new. A similar approach to judging the vital status of a patient diagnosed as "brain dead," emphasizing the crucial importance of both spontaneous breathing and the capacity for consciousness, was advocated by the late British neurologist Christopher Pallis.[8] His conceptual justification for this argument was influential in gaining acceptance for a neurological standard in the United Kingdom.*

Like this report's Position Two, Pallis attempted to strike a balance between the need to be "functionalist" and the need to remain rooted in the biological facts of total brain failure. He stated in very direct terms that the relevant functions that were irreversibly absent from the patient with a destroyed brainstem were *the ability to breathe* and *the capacity for consciousness*. When challenged as to why these two functions should be singled out, Pallis pointed to what he called "the sociological context" for basic concepts of life and death. In the West, he maintained, this context is the Judeo-Christian tradition in which "breath" and "consciousness" are two definitive features of the human soul:

> The single matrix in which my definition is embedded is a sociological one, namely Judeo-Christian culture... The "loss of the capacity for consciousness" is much the same as the "departure of the conscious soul from the body,"

---

* Other countries have adopted this conceptual framework as well. The Canadian Forum that issued its recommendations in 2006 followed the UK approach in adopting "irreversible loss of the capacity for consciousness combined with the irreversible loss of all brain stem functions, including the capacity to breathe" as the definition of neurologically determined death. Shemie, et al., "Neurological Determination of Death: Canadian Forum," S1-13.

just as "the loss of the capacity to breathe" is much the same as the "loss of the breath of life."[9]

Pallis also pointed to "the widespread identity, in various languages, of terms denoting *soul* and *breath*."[10] A challenge to this approach can be framed with two questions: First, are consciousness and breathing the *only* or the *most important* culturally significant features of the soul? And second, does this argument about traditional beliefs, bound to a particular culture, provide a sufficient rationale for a standard applicable to the transcultural, universal phenomenon of human death?

Position Two agrees with Pallis's emphasis on certain functions in preference to others, but it avoids the limitations of his approach, that is, its dependence on a particular culture. Position Two does this by taking the loss of the impulse to breathe and the total loss of engagement with the world as the cessation of the most essential functions of the organism as a whole. In this way, it builds upon an insight into biological reality, an insight latent in culture-bound notions of "breath of life" and "departure of the conscious soul from the body." It does so by articulating a philosophical conception of the biological realities of organismic life. To repeat, an organism is the unique sort of being that it is because it *can* and *must* constantly act upon and be open to its environment. From this philosophical-biological perspective, it becomes clear that a human being with a destroyed brainstem has lost the functional capacities that define organismic life.

On at least one important point, however, our Position Two and the UK neurological standard part company. The UK standard follows Pallis in accepting "death of the brainstem," rather than total brain failure, as a sufficient criterion for declaring a patient dead. Such a reduction, in addition to being conceptually suspect, is clinically dangerous because it suggests that the confirmatory tests that go beyond the bedside checks for apnea and brainstem reflexes are simply superfluous. As noted in Chapter Three, it is important to seek clarity on where a patient is on the path to the endpoint of total brain infarction. Only if the destructive cycle of infarction and swelling has reached this endpoint can the irreversibility of the patient's condition be known with confidence. Ultimately, the decision to perform these confirmatory tests (beyond those targeted at brainstem functions, for example, angiography or EEG) belongs to the attending clinician. The counsel offered here is one of caution in reaching a diagnosis with such important consequences. Only in the presence of a certain diagnosis of total brain failure do the arguments that seek to interpret this clinical finding hold weight.

ENDNOTES

[1] J. P. Lizza, "The Conceptual Basis for Brain Death Revisited: Loss of Organic Integration or Loss of Consciousness?" *Adv Exp Med Biol* 550 (2004): 52.

[2] S. Laureys, A. M. Owen, and N. D. Schiff, "Brain Function in Coma, Vegetative State, and Related Disorders," *Lancet Neurol* 3, no. 9 (2004): 537-46.

[3] H. Jonas, "Against the Stream," in *Philosophical Essays: From Ancient Creed to Technological Man* (Englewood Cliffs, NJ: Prentice-Hall, 1974), 138.

[4] D. A. Shewmon, "Chronic 'Brain Death': Meta-Analysis and Conceptual Consequences," *Neurology* 51, no. 6 (1998): 1538-45.

[5] Shewmon, "Brain and Somatic Integration," 467. Author's emphasis.

[6] Shewmon, "The Brain and Somatic Integration: Insights into the Standard Biological Rationale for Equating 'Brain Death' with Death," 457-78.

[7] Jonas, "Against the Stream," 136.

[8] C. Pallis and D. H. Harley. *ABC of Brainstem Death*. Second ed. London: BMJ Publishing Group, 1996; C. Pallis, "On the Brainstem Criterion of Death," in *The Definition of Death: Contemporary Controversies*, ed. S. J. Youngner, R. M. Arnold, and R. Schapiro (Baltimore: The Johns Hopkins University Press, 1999), 93-100.

[9] Pallis, "On the Brainstem Criterion of Death," 96.

[10] Ibid.

CHAPTER FIVE

IMPLICATIONS FOR POLICY AND PRACTICE

In this report, our fundamental question has been, *Are there adequate biological and philosophical reasons for considering patients who have suffered total brain failure to be deceased human beings?* We have sought to respond to this question in a careful, systematic fashion. In Chapter Two, we began our re-examination of the neurological standard for death by clarifying key terms. In Chapter Three, we described the condition of "total brain failure" (commonly called "brain death" or "whole brain death"), and we explored certain clinical and pathophysiological findings that were unavailable to the authors of earlier public accounts of that condition. In Chapter Four, we presented two possible answers to the central question of the report: first, a position that rejects the neurological standard for death on the grounds that it is not possible to know with certainty that an individual with total brain failure is truly dead; and second, a position that defends the neurological standard, arguing that it *is* possible to know that death has occurred in such cases. Also in Chapter Four, we sought to support this second position with a novel—and, we think, more secure—rationale. Each of the two positions has implications for policy and practice, especially with regard to organ procurement. Here in Chapter Five, we offer an analysis of these implications.

I. Rejecting the Neurological Standard: The Implications of Position One

The neurological standard for death is a well-entrenched standard, having been enshrined in law and applied in medical practice for more than two decades. To conclude now that this standard is flawed and ultimately indefensible would have serious repercussions, especially for the policy and practice of organ procurement. No patient whose heart continues beating (and whose vital organs thus remain healthy) could be declared dead; there would be no legally recognized "heart-beating cadavers." In response to such an altered approach, one of two paths could be followed: Either the link between *death* and eligibility for donation could be severed, or the law could be fashioned so that vital organs are only procured from non-heart-beating donors. Both of these possible paths require further elaboration.

A. *Severing the Link Between Death and Eligibility for Organ Donation*

The first path would entail weakening or abandoning the so-called "dead donor rule." This could be done in such a way that the same patients who are currently designated as heart-beating donors could continue to be so designated. But they would not be seen as *dead* in the eyes of the law; they would instead be described as living but "heart-beating-donation-eligible." Two steps would be required to accomplish this change.

One step would be to revise the state laws pertaining to the determination of death so that the only recognized standard would be the traditional cardiopulmonary standard. The law would then declare that only those individuals who have suffered an irreversible loss of cardiopulmonary function (spontaneous or assisted) are dead.

The other step would be to revise the anatomical gift acts that are in effect in the various states. These laws specify how individuals can express their wishes regarding organ donation if the circumstances of their death make them medically eligible. Currently, these laws uniformly stipulate that gifts of tissue, organs, or whole bodies should take effect "upon or after death."* With the suggested revision, "upon or after death" would be changed to "upon or after the point at which donation eligibility is reached." And "donation eligibility" would be defined as "the point at which, according to accepted medical standards, an individual has suffered irreversible cessation of all functions of the entire brain, including the brainstem." In other words, the language currently found in the various determination of death acts (which are modeled on the UDDA), would be transferred to the anatomical gift acts, and as a result, a patient would not need to be declared dead in order to be declared eligible for designation as a heart-beating donor.

This solution would seem to preserve the integrity of the organ procurement system by maintaining the customary boundaries between those who can be used as organ donors and those who, on ethical grounds, must be protected from such use. Moreover, it would accomplish this while setting aside the dubious claim that either clinicians or policymakers know for certain where the line between life and death is.

Despite these attractions, however, this solution is deeply disturbing, for it embraces the idea that a *living human being* may be used merely as a *means* for another human being's *ends*, losing his or her own life in the process. For good reason, many recoil from the thought that it would be permissible to end one life in order to obtain body parts needed by another. For many observers, organ transplantation as practiced today is ethically defensible precisely because only those who are *already dead* are eligible to become donors. In sum, abandoning the "dead donor rule" would entail dismantling the moral foundations of the practice of organ donation.

---

* The legality of donation from a healthy, living donor is not addressed by the anatomical gift acts. Yet the practice of living donation suggests a possible "middle course," not explored in this report, which would permit the removal of a single kidney from a donor who is *near* death—just as it is permissible for an individual to give a single kidney while alive and healthy.

This solution is worrisome on other grounds as well. Having created a category of still-living but "heart-beating-donation-eligible" individuals, we might have difficulty resisting pressure to expand the kinds of patients that could be included in that class. In fact, many who support moving away from the dead donor rule argue that such a step could be a boon to society by making *more* individuals available as heart-beating donors. If a patient need not be dead in order to be eligible for such life-ending organ donations, where would the ethical line be drawn? It has been suggested that the moral warrant for the practice could be supplied by ensuring that the would-be donor is "beyond harm."[1] In other words, the principle of non-maleficence, of "do no harm," rather than the dead donor rule, would provide the needed ethical safeguards for procuring organs from the living—for example, from patients in persistent vegetative states or from infants with anencephaly.

Yet this proposal is both conceptually suspect and practically dangerous. What exactly does "harm" mean in this context, and how do we know who is beyond harm? Might there be a temptation to interpret the class of "patients who can still be harmed" more and more narrowly in order to increase the number of donation-eligible human beings? For very sound practical reasons, the Kantian prohibition against treating living human beings merely as means and not also as ends has been fundamental to the ethics of both biomedical research and clinical medicine, at least since the promulgation of the Nuremberg Code in 1947. If that principle is worth preserving, especially in the context of organ procurement, we would do better to restrict donation-eligibility to patients who have died, as determined by clinical tests for "total brain failure," more commonly known as "whole brain death."

B. Taking Vital Organs Only from Non-Heart-Beating Donors (Controlled DCD)

In Chapter Six we shall more thoroughly explore the practice of controlled donation after cardiac death (controlled DCD), which is currently undergoing a resurgence. With this practice, organs are procured from non-heart-beating donors who have been declared dead in accordance with the traditional cardiopulmonary standard.

For those who argue that patients with total brain failure cannot, with certainty, be declared dead, controlled DCD offers a viable alternative source for much needed human organs.

Today, controlled DCD is offered as an option to families when an injured relative does not qualify to be a heart-beating donor—that is, as an opportunity to combine the generous act of organ donation with the often painful decision to forgo life-sustaining treatment for a living, but close-to-death family member. A patient diagnosed with total brain failure is considered dead by today's legal standard, and therefore eligible for organ donation immediately; but for those who regard such a patient as a still living human being, controlled DCD would be the only ethical way for that patient's organs to be donated. From this perspective, an appropriate reform might be, not to abandon the dead donor rule, but to require that *all* injured patients for whom organ donation is contemplated become asystolic before allowing organ procurement surgery to begin.

Two objections have been lodged against this approach. The first has to do with the practical consequences of this approach for organ procurement: it is likely that far fewer organs of high quality would be recovered. Because organs procured from heart-beating donors are less subject to ischemic injury, the claim is often made that obtaining such organs is a key factor in successful transplantation, especially in terms of graft survival and patient survival. In other words, organs procured from donors who have been declared dead in accordance with the traditional cardiopulmonary standard are not usually as "healthy" as those procured from heart-beating donors, nor do they last as long or permit their recipients to live as long.

Plausible as this claim might sound, however, recent studies have put it in doubt it by showing that patient and graft survival rates (at one and five years) for kidneys taken from controlled DCD donors are comparable to the rates for kidneys from heart-beating donors.[2] The same cannot be said of livers obtained by controlled DCD; graft and patient survival rates for livers recovered from controlled DCD donors are not as good as the rates for livers from heart-beating donors.[3] At this time, hearts, lungs, intestines, and pancreata are only rarely transplanted from patients whose hearts have stopped beating; thus, comparisons of these key rates are more difficult to make. In weighing these concerns about the comparative healthiness of organs from heart-beating and non-heart-beating donors, it is important to consider one possible result of restricting organ procurement to controlled DCD: such a restriction might well stimulate research into better methods of procuring and preserving organs and thereby lead to improvements in outcomes associated with organs from non-heart-beating donors.

A second objection raised against an exclusive reliance on controlled DCD as a means to procure organs concerns certain ethical and philosophical problems that we shall discuss in greater depth in Chapter Six. Here, it is important to mention that restricting organ donation to controlled DCD donors would inevitably intensify the demands on the physicians, nurses, and other health professionals responsible for such organ procurement. They would find it all the more challenging to responding, responsibly and compassionately, to concerns and needs for palliative care and family support while protecting potential donors from abuse. Such a restriction would also require wider acceptance of the idea that living individuals can and should be designated as organ donors prior to the removal of life support; in addition, the death of these donors (and the availability of their organs for transplant) would have to be more regularly declared in the expeditious way that this procedure requires.* Thus enhanced public education, discussion, and deliberation would be crucial prerequisites to any expansion of the use of controlled DCD in the ways suggested here.

---

* The concerns of various sorts of health care providers about DCD practice were surveyed in this 2006 report: M. S. Mandell, et al., "National Evaluation of Healthcare Provider Attitudes Toward Organ Donation after Cardiac Death," *Crit Care Med* 34, no. 12 (2006): 2952-8. A useful description of a conscientious program of palliative care for DCD donors and their families can be found in: C. M. Kelso, et al., "Palliative Care Consultation in the Process of Organ Donation After Cardiac Death," *J Palliat Med* 10, no. 1 (2007): 118-26.

II. Affirming the Neurological Standard: The Implications of Position Two

If the facts and arguments explored in this report lead to the conclusion that the neurological standard of whole brain death is sound on biological and philosophical grounds, then there would be no need to change the current standard of practice. Organ procurement from donors declared dead in accordance with the neurological standard would be unaffected by such a conclusion. What would be gained by this exploration, however, is a clearer understanding of the medical facts and ethical arguments supporting the practice. We review the most important of these arguments here.

First, what we have called Position Two gives a fair hearing to, and addresses on their own terms, the challenges posed by advances in the clinical and pathophysiological understanding of "brain death." To those who are troubled by doubts about the legitimacy of the neurological standard and the associated practices, Position Two should offer substantial reassurance as to the ultimate validity of the standard. To be sure, such doubts are neither entirely unwarranted nor easily dismissed. After the most serious sort of brain injury and a diagnosis of total brain failure, a patient's appearance may still engender considerable doubt as to whether he or she is dead or alive. Some of the body's systems may continue to work together in an integrated way, and it may be possible to sustain this level of functionality for an indeterminate amount of time. But such life-like appearances may fail to convey the true condition of the patient, a condition that is obscured by the artificial maintenance of breathing and circulation and the limited bodily integrity thus preserved. Many years of experience with total brain failure have revealed the truth of such a condition: the "brain-dead" patient will never recover the essential ability to interact with his or her environment that is characteristic of the living organism.

Second, a careful examination of the conceptual basis for declaring death in the midst of often confusing technological interventions invites deeper reflection on the moral obligations that we bear toward those who have crossed the threshold from life to death.

Thirty-five years ago, William F. May used the phrase, "the newly dead," to describe the bodies of those who still present the outward form of the living human beings they once were, even as mourning for their loss has already begun. As May wrote,

> The cadaver is a kind of shroud that now masks rather than expresses the soul that once animated it. And yet—while the body retains its recognizable form, even in death, it commands a certain respect. No longer a human presence, it still reminds us of that presence which once was utterly inseparable from it.[4]

To realize that death has come—even in the midst of technological interventions—is to know that the time has come to think and to act in different ways toward the newly dead human being. It is time to pay the deceased our respects, to mourn their passing—and to do so in the presence of, and with careful regard for, their mortal remains. It is also time to withhold or to withdraw such treatments as would actually constitute *mistreatment* of the newly dead. Finally, depending on the wishes of the patient and the family, it may also be time to begin the procurement of organs for the morally defensible purpose of helping the sick.

This is, perhaps, the most valuable fruit of reflecting on the foundations of today's neurological standard for death and finding them basically sound: The death of a human being is recognized for what it is, and those who survive are enabled to accept that death with finality and to regard their loved one's mortal remains with respect.

◈◈◈

ENDNOTES

[1] R. D. Truog, "Is It Time to Abandon Brain Death?" *Hastings Cent Rep* 27, no. 1 (1997): 29-37; Truog, "Too Flawed to Endure," 273-81; and S. J. Youngner and R. M. Arnold, "Philosophical Debates About the Definition of Death: Who Cares?" *J Med Philos* 26, no. 5 (2001): 527-37.

[2] See M. D. Doshi and L. G. Hunsicker, "Short- and Long-Term Outcomes with the Use of Kidneys and Livers Donated after Cardiac Death," *Am J Transplant* 7, no. 1 (2007): 122-9; J. T. Cooper et al., "Donation after Cardiac Death: The University of Wisconsin Experience with Renal Transplantation," *Am J Transplant* 4, no. 9 (2004): 1490-4; and A. M. D'Alessandro et al., "Donation after Cardiac Death: The University of Wisconsin Experience," *Ann Transplant* 9, no. 1 (2004): 68-71.

[3] See Doshi and Hunsicker, "Short and Long Term Outcomes," 122-9; P. L. Abt et al., "Survival Following Liver Transplantation from Non-Heart-Beating Donors," *Ann Surg* 239, no. 1 (2004): 87-92; and D. P. Foley et al., "Donation after Cardiac Death: The University of Wisconsin Experience with Liver Transplantation," *Ann Surg* 242, no. 5 (2005): 724-31.

[4] W. May, "Attitudes Toward the Newly Dead," *Stud Hastings Cent* 1, no. 1 (1973): 3.

CHAPTER SIX

NON-HEART-BEATING
ORGAN DONATION

O ne of the implications of rejecting the neurological standard, as we saw in Part I of Chapter Five, is that non-
heart-beating donors could become the exclusive source
of organs for procurement and transplantation. In this chapter we
examine non-heart-beating organ donation—specifically, the practice of controlled donation after cardiac death—in greater depth.

I. Background

As was noted in Chapter One, the neurological standard for the determination of death was formulated in the 1960s, in the early years
of successful cadaveric organ transplantation. Since then, the practice of transplanting organs from the dead has become
commonplace, in large measure because the "heart-beating cadaver"
has been accepted as a medical and legal reality. Heart-beating cadavers, however, are not the only source of organs from the
deceased: Human beings whose deaths have been determined according to the more traditional cardiopulmonary standard may also
provide organs. The earliest successful organ transplantations from
cadaveric donors, in fact, made use of the organs of individuals
whose deaths were determined in this way.[*]

---

[*] Two useful sources on the early use of non-heart-beating donors are M. A. De-
Vita, J. V. Snyder, and A. Grenvik, "History of Organ Donation by Patients with
Cardiac Death," *Kennedy Inst Ethics J* 3, no. 2 (1993): 113-129; and C. A. Zawis-
towski and M. A. DeVita, "Non-Heartbeating Organ Donation: A Review," *J*

A key challenge to procuring organs from non-heart-beating cadavers is posed by warm ischemic damage, caused by the lack of blood perfusion while the organs are still in the body of the newly deceased donor. To prevent or limit this damage, the time between the cessation of circulation ("effective asystole") and the procurement of organs must be minimized. For this purpose, the final cardiac contractions must be *controlled*: In the moments following asystole, the body must be prepared for surgeons either to remove the organs promptly or to maintain their viability for transplantation in the ensuing hours. For the moment of cardiac arrest to be controlled in this way, the prospective organ donor must be a patient from whom a ventilator and perhaps other forms of life-sustaining treatment will be withdrawn, either in accordance with the patient's wishes or the wishes of a surrogate. In other words, a potential non-heart-beating donor, in the vast majority of cases, is an individual who is ventilator-dependent but not yet deceased according to today's neurological standard.* The ventilator is then removed, the patient is watched and kept comfortable until the heart stops circulating blood through the body, a waiting period is observed (usually two to five minutes), and then the surgical procurement of organs begins.

Procuring organs in this way was very rare until the early 1990s—in most transplant centers throughout the United States, only heart-

---

Intensive Care Med 18, no. 4 (2003): 189-97. In addition to kidney transplantations from such cadavers in the 1950s and 1960s, the first liver transplantation in 1963 and the first heart transplant in 1967 were performed by taking the organ from a patient after life-support had been removed and the patient had become asystolic.
* Many candidates for controlled DCD are patients who are "very close to brain dead"—i.e., who are tested for total brain failure but show minimal signs of brain function that are nonetheless sufficient to preclude such a diagnosis. There are other candidates for controlled DCD, however, who are dependent on a life-sustaining technology for reasons other than a traumatic brain injury, e.g., patients with a high-spinal cord injury or patients at the end-stage of a neurodegenerative disease such as amyotrophic lateral sclerosis (ALS). For a case study of a fully conscious patient who chose to become a controlled DCD donor upon removal of the ventilator, see J. Spike, "Controlled NHBD Protocol for a Fully Conscious Person: When Death Is Intended as an End in Itself and It Has Its Own End," *J Clin Ethics* 11, no. 1 (2000): 73-7.

beating organ donors were used.[*] This restriction meant that some individuals who had suffered accidents or injuries that left them with little hope of recovery were not eligible to become donors, even if a responsible decision to remove life-sustaining interventions was made. In some cases, families who knew that their relatives wanted to be donors in the event of an accident were disappointed to find out that making this gift was not possible. This fact—along with concerns about the general shortage of available organs compared to the growing need among potential recipients— led some pioneering institutions to develop and implement non-heart-beating donor protocols.[†] These protocols codified the institutional practices for managing the withdrawal of treatment and for optimizing the conditions for organ procurement. The early controlled DCD protocols included both logistical procedures and ethical safeguards.

The work of these first institutions raised concerns among some ethicists, health care professionals, and members of the general public. For the purposes of this report, these concerns can be divided into two categories: concerns about the care of the dying patient at the end of life, and concerns about initiating organ procurement before the patient is dead. The second set of concerns is treated at length in Part II of this chapter. Regarding the first set of concerns, we shall address the principal points here while encouraging the interested reader to consult the companion volume to this white paper, *Organ Transplantation: An Ethical Inquiry by the President's Council on Bioethics*; in Chapter Three of that report, the Council offers a more thorough investigation of these concerns about care of the dying patient in the context of organ transplantation.

---

[*] One exception is the University of Wisconsin Hospital, where controlled DCD has been performed continuously since 1974. See J. Lewis, et al., "Development of the University of Wisconsin Donation after Cardiac Death Evaluation Tool," *Prog Transplant* 13, no. 4 (2003): 265-73.

[†] The first modern controlled DCD protocol was instituted at the University of Pittsburgh Medical Center in 1992. For details, see M. A. DeVita, J. V. Snyder, and A. Grenvik, "History of Organ Donation by Patients with Cardiac Death," *Kennedy Inst Ethics J* 3, no. 2 (1993): 113-29.

Those who fear that the widespread practice of controlled DCD may adversely affect the quality of care at the end of life have raised several questions, including whether families offered the option of controlled DCD are pressured to make a decision in favor of withdrawal of life support; whether the steps necessary to optimize the circumstances of death for transplant purposes interfere with good palliative care for the patient in his or her last moments; whether the family's emotional needs will be respected, considering that loved ones must be kept "out of the surgeons' way" immediately after the patient's heart stops beating; and whether the patient's death will be hastened to ensure that the procured organs are maximally viable.[*]

In response to such concerns, institutions seeking to expand their transplant programs to include non-heart-beating donors have incorporated ethical safeguards into their transplantation protocols. To aid institutions in the development of ethically sound protocols, two reports by the Institute of Medicine on non-heart-beating donation were published.[1] The Society for Critical Care Medicine also published an analysis of the issue, detailing the requirements for the practice to be carried out in an ethically sound manner.[2] More recently, a report was published by a National Conference on Donation After Cardiac Death.[3] This report, while supportive of the practice, addressed medical and ethical concerns that have

---

[*] Some detail about this last concern: The patient who is designated a candidate for controlled DCD must not only be ventilator-dependent, but also likely to expire (become asystolic) within a short window of time after removal of the ventilator. The longer a patient removed from ventilation "lingers" before expiring, the more likely are the organs destined for transplantation to be damaged by warm ischemia. Institutional protocols specify the maximum time—generally between thirty minutes and two hours—that a patient removed from ventilation can linger before the organs are judged to be no longer viable, For a description of a technique used to estimate how long a particular patient will take to expire (and, thus, whether he or she can be a candidate for controlled DCD) see Lewis, et al., "Development," 265-73. Concerns about the temptation to hasten death stem from the fact that hopes are raised and many expensive preparations are made on the expectation that death will occur quickly enough to allow procurement of transplantable organs.

arisen as more institutions have started to procure organs in this way.

The practice of controlled DCD has expanded rapidly in the last decade. In 1997, for example, there were seventy-eight cases of organ procurement from DCD donors; in 2007, there were 793 cases. In 1997, only six organ procurement organizations (OPOs) reported five or more controlled DCD procurements within their respective areas; in 2007, forty-one OPOs reported five or more controlled DCD procurements.[4] This expansion has been aided by requirements from such national bodies as the United Network for Organ Sharing (UNOS) and the Joint Commission (formerly the Joint Commission on Accreditation of Healthcare Organizations or JCAHO) that hospitals either institute controlled DCD protocols or, at the very least, address the practice in their statement of hospital policy.[5]

II. The Rush to Declare Death and the Problem of Irreversibility

Are those who donate organs under a controlled DCD protocol actually dead at the time of donation? It might seem somewhat surprising that this is a matter of controversy. After all, at the time of procurement, the donor's heart has stopped and he or she is no longer breathing—either spontaneously or with ventilator support. Thus, the individual would seem to meet the first (more traditional) standard for determining death, that is, in the wording of the UDDA, "irreversible cessation of circulatory and respiratory functions."

The difficulty here stems from the crucial requirement that cessation of circulatory and respiratory functions be *irreversible*. In truth, there is reason to doubt that the cessation of circulatory and respiratory functions is irreversible, in the strict sense, in every case of controlled DCD. To call the loss of functions irreversible, it must be the case that the functions could not possibly return, either on their own or with external help. It is often possible, however, to cause circulation and respiration to return by administering cardiopulmonary resuscitation (CPR). If this were attempted after the "declaration of death" in controlled DCD, some patients would indeed regain—for a brief time, at least—a heartbeat and some capacity to breathe. If this were to occur, the patient would certainly not have been "resurrected," but instead would have been (according to the cardiopulmonary standard of death) resuscitated, i.e., prevented from dying. Thus, the prior "declaration of death" would turn out to be questionable. The patient was, it could be argued, no more dead than a person who collapses in his or her home, loses heartbeat, and is resuscitated by paramedics who arrive moments later.

It is important to note that this hypothetical scenario of resuscitating a patient who has been prepared for a controlled DCD procurement is merely a "thought experiment." In reality, attempting to revive such a patient would be ruled out ethically because the practice of controlled DCD is premised on the assumption that the individual's family has decided to allow withdrawal of life-sustaining interventions and would, therefore, want to abstain from any efforts to prevent the patient's death (perhaps by consenting to a "do not resuscitate" order). For this reason, many have argued that the word "irreversible" in this context should be understood in a weaker sense than that spelled out above: It should be understood to mean "cessation of circulatory and respiratory functions under conditions in which those functions cannot return on their own and *will not* be restored by medical interventions."[*] This looser sense of the term "irreversible" would seem to be a better fit in this context.

The problem of ascertaining irreversibility in controlled DCD procurement is illustrated by a series of procurements and transplants

---

[*] See, for instance, S. J. Youngner, R. M. Arnold, and M. A. DeVita, "When Is 'Dead'?" *Hastings Cent Rep* 29, no. 6 (1999): 14-21. For the purposes of the argument made here, it is assumed that two to five minutes of waiting time is enough to guarantee that the heart will not auto-resuscitate, i.e., that it will not begin to beat again on its own. There is insufficient scientific evidence to decide whether this assumption is always justified, as has been noted by many commentators, including the National Conference on Donation After Cardiac Death. See J. L. Bernat, et al., "Report of a National Conference on Donation after Cardiac Death," *Am J Transplant* 6, no. 2 (2006): 282.

carried out in Denver, Colorado, between 2004 and 2007.[6] In each of the three procurements conducted under a controversial controlled DCD protocol, the heart was taken from a severely brain-injured (but not "brain dead") infant whose family had authorized removal of life-sustaining treatments. In one case, the procurement team waited three minutes after cardiac contractions had stopped before removing the heart from the donor. In the other two cases, they waited only seventy-five seconds—a shorter time than either the Society of Critical Care Medicine or the National Conference on Donation After Cardiac Death has recommended.[7] In each of the three cases, the hearts were transplanted and the recipients were still alive six months post-transplant.

In analyzing these controversial cases, it is important to note that the fact that the recipients of these hearts were restored to a state of health does do not imply that the donors' conditions were anything less than terminal and dire. To state this another way, the *heart*, itself, in each of these cases, was healthy enough to become an effective organ again in the body of the recipient, even though the overall condition of the body of the dying donor made it impossible for the donor's health to be restored.

The ethically troubling point is brought into sharp relief when we think of the moment of procurement. In each case, the heart of the infant had stopped. But was the infant actually dead? Because the heart tissue itself was not beyond the point of resuscitation once transferred to the recipient, it is clear that (as in some other controlled DCD cases) the cessation of cardiac function in these infants *might have been reversed*, albeit only for a short time, had there been a desire to do so. What prevented this from occurring was not a certainty that resuscitation attempts on the would-be donor would fail, but rather the decision made by the parents that no effort to resuscitate should be made. In short, the donor had only suffered "irreversible cessation of circulatory and respiratory functions," if the term "irreversible" is taken in the weaker sense that Youngner and others have proposed.

In any event, such debates about the proper meaning of "irreversible" do not address a more pressing ethical dilemma—the question of whether there is something wrong with *rushing* to make a determination of death because of external pressures to procure organs as expeditiously as possible. There is reason to worry that this practice—if carried out on a wide scale—could make the donor's death seem like a mere formality, with "patient dies" becoming simply another item to check off on a list of events required for a successful controlled DCD procurement.

There might be something to learn about this ethical concern from anecdotes of physicians who are called upon to declare death in more routine hospital cases. It is said that experienced physicians will take their time in proceeding to the patient's room to declare him or her dead. They may even deliberately linger to give the patient's body ample time to complete the dying process. This is not done, we can imagine, because of a lack of confidence in the physician's own judgment, but rather out of a sense that, in approaching the mysterious threshold between life and death, circumspection and caution are required. Rushing to make a declaration as quickly as possible is not viewed as respectful or appropriate. Unfortunately, such a deliberate demeanor is harder to maintain if the death is going to be "made use of" for the sake of other needy patients.

Health professionals should help families understand that the process of mourning their loved ones is likely to be disrupted by a controlled DCD protocol and that this disruption is part of the sacrifice they are making in giving their loved ones' organs to the sick. They should also help families understand the controversies about "irreversibility" that will always be a part of controlled DCD procurement. In addition to such steps that should be taken on a case by case basis, there ought to be a broader public discussion and debate about the propriety of controlled DCD as a standard practice in hospitals. With the spread of controlled DCD practice to more and more hospitals, it is clear that patients and their families will need to come to terms with this still novel aspect of end-of-life decision making.

The integrity of the procurement system has just as much at stake in the context of controlled DCD procurements as it has in the context of procurements made after diagnoses of total brain failure.

The clinical preference for acquiring the most viable organs possible cannot be allowed to undermine the principle that death should be declared only when there are sound medical reasons to do so. In light of this, more research should be done to investigate the question of auto-resuscitation (mentioned in the footnote on page 84). The assurance that the heart will not restart on its own within the relevant time frame, combined with an informed decision by the patient and family in favor of controlled DCD, may or may not be *sufficient* as a moral warrant for declaring death, but it is certainly *necessary*. Again, the principle here is clear: Death should be declared on the sole basis of the medical facts of the patient's case. Since ruling out the possibility of auto-resuscitation is an essential step here—a point that has been emphasized by the IOM, the Society of Critical Care Medicine, and others—the prediction must be based on sound and publicly available evidence.

ENDNOTES

[1] Institute of Medicine, *Non-Heart-Beating Organ Transplantation: Medical and Ethical Issues in Procurement* (Washington, D.C.: National Academy Press, 1997); and Institute of Medicine, *Non-Heart-Beating Organ Transplantation: Practice and Protocols* (Washington, D.C.: National Academy Press, 2000).

[2] Society of Critical Care Medicine, "Recommendations for Nonheartbeating Organ Donation," *Crit Care Med* 29, no. 9 (2001): 1826-31.

[3] J. L. Bernat et al., "Report of a National Conference on Donation after Cardiac Death," *Am J Transplant* 6, no. 2 (2006): 281-91.

[4] Institute of Medicine, *Organ Donation: Opportunities for Action* (Washington, D.C.: National Academy Press, 2006), 142-43; Kevin O'Connor, Senior Vice-President, New England Organ Bank, Personal Communication, September 12, 2008.

[5] For Joint Commission requirement, see Joint Commission, "2009 Accreditation Requirements: Accreditation Program: Critical Access Hospital," (2008), Standard TS.01.01.01, Element 4. Available online at http://www.jointcommission.org/ NR/rdonlyres/8093C734-2317-4CDC-A0BF-BFB2DF0FBAD1/0/CAH_All Chapters.pdf (accessed Sept.12, 2008). For UNOS requirement, see Appendix B to UNOS Bylaws, available online at http://www.unos.org/policiesandBylaws2/ bylaws/UNOSByLaws/pdfs/bylaw_31.pdf (accessed Sept. 12, 2008).

[6] M. M. Boucek et al., "Pediatric Heart Transplantation after Declaration of Cardiocirculatory Death," *N Engl J Med* 359, no. 7 (2008): 709-14.

[7] Society of Critical Care Medicine, "Recommendations for Nonheartbeating Organ Donation," 1826-31; and J. L. Bernat et al., "Report of a National Conference on Donation after Cardiac Death," 281-91.

CHAPTER SEVEN

A SUMMARY OF THE COUNCIL'S DEBATE ON THE NEUROLOGICAL STANDARD FOR DETERMINING DEATH

As we noted in the Preface and in Chapter One, although this report addresses several controversies in the determination of death, including those arising in the context of controlled DCD, its primary focus is on the debates surrounding the neurological standard for the determination of death. In its deliberations, the President's Council on Bioethics did, indeed, discuss controlled DCD and the traditional cardiopulmonary standard; it also voiced concerns about the problem of ensuring adequate end-of-life care for the patient-donor. The Council's principal concern, however, was with the question, *Does a diagnosis of "whole brain death" mean that a human being is dead?* In other words, does the neurological standard rest on a sound biological and philosophical basis?

Among members of the President's Council on Bioethics, the prevailing opinion is that the current neurological standard for declaring death, grounded in a careful diagnosis of total brain failure, is biologically and philosophically defensible. The ethical controversies explored in this report were first raised for the Council during its inquiry into organ transplantation: as most deceased organ donors have been declared dead on the basis of the neurological standard, questions about its validity have an obvious relevance for organ procurement. The Council concluded that, despite that connection, the two matters—determining death and procuring organs—should be addressed separately. More precisely, questions about the vital status of neurologically injured individuals

89

should be taken up *prior to* and *apart from* ethical issues in organ procurement from deceased donors.

Two such questions must be posed and answered in light of certain clinical and pathophysiological facts and in light of the competing interpretations of those facts. First, *are patients in the condition of total brain failure actually dead?* And, second, *can we answer the first question with sufficient certainty to ground a course of action that treats the body in that condition as the mortal remains of a human being?* Most members of the Council have concluded that both questions can and should be answered in the affirmative. They reaffirm and support the well-established dictates of both law and practice in this area.

Many members of the Council, however, judge that affirmative answers to these questions must be supported by arguments better than and different from those offered in the past. Until now, two facts about the diagnosis of total brain failure have been taken to provide fundamental support for a declaration of death: first, that the body of a patient with this diagnosis is no longer a "somatically integrated whole," and, second, that the ability of the patient to maintain circulation will cease within a definite span of time. Both of these supposed facts have been persuasively called into question in recent years.

Another argument, however, can be advanced to support the declaration of death following a diagnosis of total brain failure. It is one that many members of the Council find both sound and persuasive, for it appeals to long recognized facts about the condition of total brain failure, while doing so in a way that is both novel and philosophically convincing. According to this argument, the patient with total brain failure is no longer able to carry out the fundamental work of a living organism. Such a patient has lost—and lost irreversibly—a fundamental openness to the surrounding environment as well as the capacity and drive to act on this environment on his or her own behalf. As described in Chapter Four, a living organism engages in self-sustaining, need-driven activities critical to and constitutive of its commerce with the surrounding world. These activities are authentic signs of active and ongoing life. When these signs are absent, and these activities have ceased, then a judgment that the organism as a whole has died can be made with confidence. However, another view of the neurological standard was also voiced within the Council. According to this view, there can be no certainty about the vital status of patients with total brain failure; hence, the only prudent and defensible conclusion is that such patients are severely injured—but not yet dead—human beings. Therefore, only the traditional signs—irreversible cessation of heart and lung function—should be used to declare a patient dead. Also, according to this view, medical interventions for patients with total brain failure should be withdrawn only after they have been judged to be *futile*, in the sense of medically *ineffective and non-beneficial* to the patient and disproportionately *burdensome*. Such a judgment must be made on ethical grounds that consider the whole situation of the particular patient and not merely the biological facts of the patient's condition.* Once such a judgment has been made, interventions can and should be withdrawn so that the natural course of the patient's injury can reach its inevitable terminus. Only after this process has occurred and the patient's heart has stopped beating, is there a morally valid warrant to proceed with such steps as preparation for burial or for organ procurement.

With this report, the President's Council on Bioethics seeks to shed light on a matter of ongoing ethical and philosophical controversy in contemporary medicine. Knowing when death has come, along

---

* This understanding of medical futility has been developed in several papers by Edmund D. Pellegrino, the Council's chairman. In these (as well as other) works, Pellegrino argues that clinical judgments of the futility of a given therapeutic intervention involve a "judicious balancing" of three factors: (1) the *effectiveness* of the given intervention, which is an objective determination that physicians alone can make; (2) the *benefit* of that intervention, which is an assessment that only patients and/or their surrogates can make; and (3) the *burdens* of the intervention (e.g., the cost, discomfort, pain, or inconvenience), which are jointly assessed by both physicians and patients and/or their surrogates. For example, see E. D. Pellegrino, "Decisions to Withdraw Life-Sustaining Treatment: A Moral Algorithm," *JAMA*, 283, no. 8 (2000): 1065-7; and E. D. Pellegrino, "Futility in Medical Decisions: The Word and the Concept," *HEC Forum*, 17, no. 4 (2005): 308-18.

with what can and should be done before and after it has arrived, has always been a problem for humankind, to one degree or another. But the nature and significance of the problem have changed over time, especially in the wake of technological advances that enable us to sustain life, or perhaps just the appearance of it, indefinitely. Given these changes and others that are yet to come, the Council believes that it is necessary and desirable to re-examine our ideas and practices concerning the human experience of death in light of new evidence and novel arguments. Undertaken in good faith, such a re-examination is a responsibility incumbent upon all who wish to keep human dignity in focus, especially in the sometimes disorienting context of contemporary medicine.

PERSONAL STATEMENTS

PERSONAL STATEMENT OF ALFONSO GÓMEZ–LOBO, DR. PHIL.

The purpose of this statement is to present my personal views on three different issues that arise within the debate addressed in the present report.

Conceptual Issues

Since the publication of the reports by the Harvard Ad Hoc Committee (1968) and by the President's Commission (1981), it has become commonplace to claim that "the definition of death" has been revised, and that, accordingly, the definition "has changed" or "has evolved." It is thus suggested that the medical profession now has an understanding of death that is different from the one it had a few decades ago. Moreover, the "new definition," the one that "defines" death as "whole brain death," is the one that has been enshrined in the law.

In my view, this use of the philosophical term "definition" is inaccurate and all too often seriously misleading.

To define a term is to provide, in other words, an account of its meaning. Thus, if we define "triangle" as "a plane figure with three straight sides" and the definition is changed to "a plane figure with four straight sides," then the term "triangle" will no longer single out triangles, but squares. In fact, a change in definition usually entails a change in reference. Hence, if the definition of "death" changes, we will not be referring to the same natural phenomenon we had been trying to identify before the semantic change took place.

If the contemporary dispute about death is to be intelligible, the definition of "death" must remain stable.

A long tradition in philosophy with many contemporary defenders points out that there are two kinds of definitions: ordinary language definitions and specialized language definitions. Most people understand "water" to mean, roughly, "a transparent liquid that flows from the kitchen or bathroom faucet, and is safe to drink." However, people with some knowledge of chemistry define it as "a liquid whose basic molecule is composed of two atoms of hydrogen and one of oxygen."

Likewise, it is reasonable to expect that there will be two kinds of definition for the term "death." First, "death" as ordinarily understood means "the irreversible cessation of life" and applies to all things that have been alive. There is no separate definition that applies, say, only to humans, to the exclusion of animals or plants. Nor can life irreversibly cease more than once. Hence, there is only one death for each organism. Death, furthermore, is a natural, biological event with social consequences, not a moral, legal, or political decision on the part of those observing it. Death itself should not be confused with the ruling that death has occurred.

The definition of "death" as "the irreversible cessation of life" is a definition by exclusion. It is a derivative account that is parasitic on the more primitive notion of life. A second, specialized language definition of "death" would thus have to specify, in the language of biology, the essential properties of life. Although progress has been made in the understanding of DNA and other driving factors of life, we are far from being able to give an essential definition of "life" analogous to the H_2O definition of "water." We must resort instead to the observable signs of life. These allow us to state whether an organism is alive or dead. If a body is able to process nutrition, eliminate waste, and exhibit proportional growth, homeostasis, etc., and, moreover, it engages in these functions in an integrated manner, we shall correctly deem it to be alive. If it fails to do this, and starts to decompose and disintegrate, we will rightly judge it to be dead.

In judging as we have just described, we have adopted observable criteria for life. "Criteria" is the plural of "criterion," a word whose Greek roots suggest the idea of separation or distinction. A good example of a criterion is a sieve that separates liquids from solids. A criterion is thus chosen, and is sometimes even man-made. We decide what we will use as a criterion, that is, as an instrument for setting apart the living from the dead. An alternative, synonymous expression commonly used to refer to criteria is the word "standards."

Thus, the appeal to the traditional cardiorespiratory criterion or standard is a choice to determine death by verifying the irreversible cessation of heartbeat and breathing. To choose to determine death by total brain failure does not change the definition of death. It is a decision to use a different standard to determine death.

A standard is chosen, but the choice can be wrong. It depends on what the function of the standard is expected to be. If the goal is to separate liquids from sand, a sieve with large holes will be the wrong choice. Likewise, if a criterion to determine death is chosen that leads us to declare dead certain individuals who continue to display the observable signs of life, then that standard will have been wrongly chosen.

The "higher brain death" criterion or standard for death seems to be a wrong choice for several reasons: it turns on an unpersuasive distinction between the death of plants or animals, and the death of a person. Moreover, it requires us to assume that we undergo two deaths: the death of the mind and the death of the body (although for most people they would be simultaneous events). Furthermore, it leaves behind not a cadaver, but an ostensibly living body.

The choice of a specific criterion or standard is insufficient, by itself, to determine whether someone is dead or alive. A trained, experienced eye must observe whether the conditions specified in the formulation of the standard are or are not objectively present in a patient. To satisfy this diagnostic need, tests are designed to operate under each of the different criteria. To place a stethoscope on the chest of a patient in order to verify whether his or her heart has stopped beating is to conduct a test under the cardiorespiratory standard. To perform an EEG is to conduct one of the tests to establish total brain failure.

Tests can be inaccurate and lead to unclear results, that is, to the conclusion that we are uncertain whether someone is dead or alive.[1] The inaccuracy of tests can also lead to false results, such as declaring dead someone who later recovers. The epistemic question of whether we can be certain that someone is dead or alive leads to further refinement of our tests, and may play a crucial role in reaching a moral judgment, but it should not be confused with the physiological question—whether the brain is the organ responsible for the integrated functioning of the organism, so that total brain failure is the same as the irreversible cessation of the life of a given organism.

Physiological Issues

During the discussion of the present report, evidence was offered that seems to show that survival after total brain failure is not only possible, but has been documented in approximately 175 cases. This would entail "that the body's integrative unity derives from mutual interaction among its parts, not from a top-down imposition of one 'critical organ' upon an otherwise mere bag of organs and tissues."[2]

In order to disprove this last finding, one (or both) of the following two conditions would have to be met:

First, that the "brain dead" individuals who continue to live are not really "brain dead." That is, they would all have to be cases of misdiagnosis of total and irreversible brain failure. Given the evidence adduced (especially the results of a brain autopsy of a patient who survived twenty years after the diagnosis of total brain failure due to bacterial meningitis),[3] it seems to me that there are credible reasons to think that the patients were indeed "brain dead."

And second, that the functions exhibited by the patients are not indicative of the integrated functioning of an organism. In other words, one would have to argue that all observed biological processes were only lingering activations of some subsystems of the body: the body as a whole would not be alive because of its lack of holistic properties. This last claim is contradicted by the fact that, for example, proportional growth and, more generally, homeostasis, and perhaps other observable phenomena, cannot be explained as the isolated functioning of a part of the organism. I think it is reasonable to think that these are holistic properties that involve the organism as a whole.

On the basis of the aforementioned findings, I am inclined to hold that the choice of whole brain failure as a standard for death is a questionable choice, whether it is based on the physiological claim that the brain is the integrative organ for the whole organism or on the general biological claim that the spontaneous drive to breathe, which is dependent on the brain, is necessary for life. The existence of conscious, yet apneic, patients allows us to dispose of the latter claim. Since some apneic individuals are alive, it follows that it appears to be false that all individuals who lack the drive to breathe spontaneously are dead.

With regard to the role of the brain, there is a further physiological consideration to be taken into account. During the early embryonic stages of an organism, there is certainly integrated functioning of subsystems, and this happens before the brain is formed. This suggests that the brain is not the organ that is responsible for the integrated functioning of the organism of which it is a part, but rather that it is itself a product of a prior dynamism of the integrated whole.

From the information presented to me, I am provisionally inclined to side with what in the report is called Position One. I am aware of its minority status, and that it could be overthrown if new evidence shows that either alleged "whole brain dead" patients have been misdiagnosed or that the apparent survival of those patients is only a lingering preservation of uncoordinated physiological subsystems.

Ethical Issues

In my view, the ethical cornerstone of vital organ transplantation is the dead donor rule: no one should be intentionally killed so that his or her organs may benefit someone else. To violate this rule is to go against the goals of medicine and to violate a basic norm of human interaction.

If a certain standard or criterion, no matter how widely accepted, entails the risk of violating the dead donor rule, then it should be revised in light of the empirical evidence. If it turns out that the current neurological standard allows, in certain cases, the extraction of organs from individuals who are still alive, then the morally right thing to do would be to abandon it and adopt a safer criterion.

ENDNOTES

[1] K. G. Karakatsanis. "'Brain Death': Should It Be Reconsidered?" *Spinal Cord* 46, no. 6 (2008): 396-401.

[2] D. A. Shewmon. "Chronic 'Brain Death': Meta-Analysis and Conceptual Consequences." *Neurology* 51, no. 6 (1998): 1538-45.

[3] S. Repertinger, W. P. Fitzgibbons, M. F. Omojola, and R. A. Brumback. "Long Survival Following Bacterial Meningitis-Associated Brain Destruction." *J Child Neurol* 21, no. 7 (2006): 591-5

PERSONAL STATEMENT OF GILBERT C. MEILAENDER, PH.D.

I write to underscore a few matters that are, I think, important aspects of this white paper's discussion of controversies in the determination of death.

(1) The Council rejects the view that the criteria for determining death should be shaped or determined by our need and desire for transplantable organs. We should not create "legal fictions" or "social agreements" whose aim is less an accurate determination of death than a ready supply of organs. Whatever else human beings may be, they are living bodies, and their death is a biological reality that we need to mark as accurately as we are able.

(2) This does not mean, however, that the determination of death is a straightforwardly empirical matter. In order to know when a biological organism—and, in particular, a complicated one such as a human being—has died, we need as much philosophical clarity as we can manage about what makes a human being a living whole. Hence, this document does more than just consider medical and biological facts; it also develops a theory of what makes an organism a living organism.

(3) This theory is, I believe, the most significant contribution of the white paper. For decades now the determination of death in many cases—and especially in cases where organs have then been taken for transplant—has been made on the basis of a neurological standard (commonly referred to as "brain death," but in this document called "total brain failure"). The rationale offered in support of that standard has been that a body which has suffered irreversible loss of all brain activity (which has lost, so to speak, its "executive" power) can no longer function as an integrated whole and hence is

no longer a living whole. This rationale was never entirely persuasive and has become even less so over time. The Council offers here (in Position Two of Chapter Four) what is, in my view, a more adequate rationale for continued use of a neurological standard in the determination of death: a philosophical rationale that seeks to characterize the fundamental work of self-preservation which any living organism must carry out if it is to remain alive.

(4) Chapter Four develops this rationale with admirable succinctness and clarity, and there is no need for me to repeat it. I do, however, want to emphasize that the capacities which characterize the work by which an organism sustains itself (openness to the surrounding environment, ability to act upon that environment, and inner experience of need) may be present even when a human being is no longer conscious of self or of the surrounding world. Consciousness is a prominent mode of a living human being's openness to the world, but not the only mode. Its presence is sufficient to assure us that a human being still lives. But even its permanent absence is not sufficient evidence of death, for a human being may have permanently lost (so far as we can tell) all capacity for consciousness while continuing to be a living organism in the terms Position Two sets forth. A permanently unconscious human being who breathes spontaneously manifests openness to the surrounding environment in its need for oxygen, acts upon that environment by breathing to take in the oxygen it needs, and manifests an inner drive to breathe. Such a person is surely severely disabled, but is not dead.

(5) A drive to breathe, moved by one's own inner impulse, is—as Position Two notes—not the same as "being ventilated." A coordinated exchange of oxygen and carbon dioxide still takes place in a body whose work of breathing has been replaced by mechanical ventilation, but this exchange "is not the achievement of the organism or a sign of its vitality." Nevertheless, the bodies of human beings who have suffered total brain failure (and, hence, are dead according to the rationale provided by Position Two) may, if ventilated, still exhibit some characteristics that suggest continued life. This fact has led some to reject not only the rationale currently used to justify a neurological standard for death (i.e., loss of bodily inte-

gration), but also the notion that death can be determined on the basis of neurological injury, apart from the familiar signs of stopped heartbeat and circulation. These critics hold that death must be determined as it was before mechanical ventilators and the concept of "brain death" came upon the scene—namely by observing irreversible loss of heart and lung activity (and this view is developed in Position One of Chapter Four). Were this critique accepted, it would, of course, create complications for organ transplantation, since there would no longer be "brain dead" but still ventilated "cadavers" from whom organs could be taken. These complications alone, however, cannot be reason to reject such a view.

(6) Although I take this critique seriously, it has not persuaded me that we must abandon a (suitably articulated) neurological standard for determining death. The critics who adopt Position One are still overly tied to the language of somatic integration. That is not unimportant, of course, but it does not get to the heart of what makes an organism living. So, for example, there is a difference between the drive of hunger, which turns an organism toward its environment in search of the means of its self-preservation, and the transfer of nutrients in a body—and a difference between the drive to breathe and the exchange of gases in a body. In each case the former is the mark of a living being, the latter something more like a mechanical process that does not indicate the being's own attempt to engage its world. Hence, my own view is that we have good reason to adopt the rationale developed in Position Two, a rationale that justifies us in using a neurological standard to determine death. I say this not because I think organ transplantation unproblematic; I do not. I say it only because it seems to me an accurate account of what we mean when we distinguish between the living and the dead.

⚬⚬

PERSONAL STATEMENT OF
EDMUND D. PELLEGRINO, M.D.

The Chairman's first obligation concerning any Council report is to ensure that it fairly and accurately reflects the opinions of the Council members and that the evidence and research supporting those opinions is complete and reliably presented. Having participated personally in the preparation of this white paper, I believe it satisfies those conditions.

Like any Council member, the Chairman is free to express his personal views on the debated issues. To that end, I offer my own interpretations of some of the evidence and arguments employed in the white paper. I do so in the spirit of "good faith" urged in the white paper's closing exhortation "...to re-examine the human experience of death in light of new evidence and novel argument."

After extended deliberation, the Council made these recommendations: (1) to reaffirm the ethical propriety of the "dead donor rule" (DDR); (2) to reaffirm the ethical acceptability of the neurological standard (total brain failure, including the brain stem) as well as the cardiopulmonary standard (irreversible cessation of both cardiac and respiratory functions); and (3) to reject the use of patients in permanent vegetative states as organ donors.

I am in general agreement with these recommendations, but I differ with some of the arguments advanced for them. This contribution focuses on four issues: (1) the matter of definitions, (2) the significance of the DDR, (3) the relative merits of the neurological and cardiopulmonary standards, and (4) the places of prudential reasoning and futility in remedying some of the problems with both standards.

The Matter of "Definition"

The so-called "definitions" of death fall into two categories: the philosophical and the empirical. The first seek a conceptual under-standing of the essential differences between life and death. The second seek to determine the clinical signs, tests, or criteria which separate life and death most accurately. Ideally, a full definition would link the concept of life (or death) with its clinical manifesta-tions as closely as possible. So far, this linkage has been the subject of controversy because of its pivotal role in ethically justifying the removal of vital organs from donors in transplantation protocols.

Philosophical "Definitions"

My colleague, Professor Gómez-Lobo, in his personal commentary, outlines the requirements for a philosophically valid definition of death and the failure of present attempts at definition to satisfy those requirements. I agree with Professor Gómez-Lobo's analysis. Here, I need only remind us about the difficulties inherent in all definitions. As Aristotle would have it: "Clearly, then, a definition is the easiest of all things to demolish, while to establish one is the hardest."[1] As the debates in this white paper attest, this is especially true for so-called definitions of death and life. Each is defined in terms of the absence of the other. Rather than being defined con-ceptually, each is identified with a set of empirically observable criteria.

Shortly after the proposal of the Harvard criteria for total brain death was advanced, the philosopher Hans Jonas described the cen-tral philosophical difficulty in this way:

> Reality of certain kinds—of which the life-death spectrum is perhaps only one—may be imprecise in itself, or the knowledge obtainable of it may be. To acknowledge such a state of affairs is more adequate to it than a precise defi-nition which does violence to it. I am challenging the undue precision of a definition and its application to an imprecise field.[2]

On Jonas's view, the intrinsic connection between the empirical re-alities of biological death and its conceptual formulation is too weak to support the moral weight required to justify removal of vital or-gans. Jonas recognizes the logical fact that states of imprecision in our perception of reality cannot give rise to precision in our con-cept of reality. Similarly, states of doubt cannot give rise to certitude.

Aristotle issues the same kind of warning when making ethical judgments:

> Our discussion will be adequate if it has as much clearness as the subject matter admits of, for precision is not to be sought for alike in all discussions, any more than in all the products of the crafts.[3]

This warning is especially relevant for any attempt to arrive at moral judgments in the presence of reasonable doubt about the clinical criteria for death.

These same criticisms apply to proposed philosophical definitions of death in the absence of indisputable objective signs of death. Four such attempts to define death in philosophical terms are con-sidered, i.e., loss of integrative functioning of the whole organism, failure to engage the environment spontaneously by respiration, loss of consciousness and sentiency, and the separation of some vital principle from the body.

Integrative Functions: Loss of somatic integration of the organism as a whole as a result of brain death was proposed nearly thirty years ago by the then-President's Commission.[4] In recent years, this criterion has been cast into doubt by a long series of clinical observations. A list, from the work of neurologist Alan Shewmon, is presented in Chapter Four of the white paper.[5] Strenuously debated in the past, the criterion of somatic integration enjoys waning support today.[6]

Engagement with the Environment: The Council's white paper proffers a more attractive, philosophical argument, i.e., loss of the capacity by the apneic patient for active spontaneous engagement with the environment through the function of breathing. The patient lacking this capacity is said to be "dead," even if respiratory function and cell metabolism are sustained by mechanical ventilation because they are not, then, the result of "spontaneous" respiration. However, other patients kept alive "artificially"—by pacemakers, defibrillators, vasopressors, ventricular assist devices, artificial nutrition and hydration, etc.—are not, by that fact alone, considered to be "dead." Patients with respiratory paralysis due to poliomyelitis or cervical spine trans-section have lived with the assistance of respirators for many years. Few would embalm or bury these supposed "living cadavers" before their hearts had stopped irreversibly.

Loss of Sentience and Mental Capacity: Some have proposed a philosophical definition of death based in total loss of conscious mental capacity. Mental capacity, it is argued, is a fundamental capability specific to human life. If it is completely lost, it is argued, the subject is no longer entitled to the moral status of a member of the natural kind we call "human." "A human body that can only function biologically without inward mental life does not sustain a moral agent."[7] This argument, again, identifies death of the organism with death of one organ —the brain. The sufficiency of the proposed criteria for "death" of the brain is, however, precisely what is currently being debated.

Separation of Soul and Body: Finally, the metaphysical definition of death as separation of the body from its vital principle is still held as the authoritative definition by many worldwide. Plato put it most bluntly: "Death in my opinion is nothing else but the separation from each other of two things, soul and body."[8] No precise congruence of this concept with any observable set of clinical facts has ever been agreed upon.

In the end, attempts at philosophical definitions lack the empirical precision required for a definition, as Jonas has pointed out. Until an empirically sound criterion for death is found, the lack of a conjunction between concept and reality remains a problem. Most such attempts now end in some form of circular reasoning—defining death in terms of life and life in terms of death without a true "definition" of one or the other. Plato recognized the circular reasoning in this way: "….about life and death, do you not admit that death is the opposite of life?"[9]

Each philosophical definition builds on clinical criteria that are still debated. While *necessary*, these criteria are not *sufficient per se* to define death. The search must continue for better physiological criteria if there is to be satisfactory closure of the gap between philosophical concepts and clinical reality.

The only indisputable signs of death are those we have known since antiquity, i.e., loss of sentience, heartbeat, and breathing; mottling and coldness of the skin; muscular rigidity; and eventual putrefaction as the result of generalized autolysis* of body cells.[10] There is no biomarker to tell us when this trajectory begins. Instead, we make judgments that the process of autolysis is underway with sufficient certainty to embalm, dissect, cremate, mourn, and bury the body long before signs of putrefaction are evident.

The possibilities of organ transplantation have forced us to shorten the time for observation and deliberation in the interests of preserving the vitality of organs to be transplanted. In place of a prudent waiting period, we must declare a donor to be dead as soon as possible, by one or the other of two standards, both of which are subject to increasing uncertainty about their validity. Most of this debate is covered extensively in the Council's forthcoming report on organ transplantation. Allusion here will be made only to the comparative reliability of the neurological and the cardiopulmonary standards.

Preserving the "Dead Donor Rule"

The DDR has been the anchor for the moral and social acceptability of organ transplantation protocols from their earliest days. This rule requires assurance of the death of the donor as the first step in

---

* "The destruction of cells of the body by the action of their own enzymes." OED.

any ethically legitimate transplantation protocol (other than those involving healthy, living donors). In addition, the death of the patient must not be hastened, nor end of life care compromised in any way, to accommodate transplantation protocols. No protocol can claim moral sanction without fidelity to this rule.

Today, as serious doubts about the reliability of brain death criteria and the neurological standard persist, some bioethicists are proposing modification or even abolition of the DDR. Robert Truog and Franklin Miller hold that since both the brain death and cardiac death criteria have "...never been fully convincing," the only ethically valid precondition for transplantation is the consent of the donor or his or her surrogates prior to the withdrawal of life support.[11] Robert Veatch also doubts the reliability of both the neurological and the cardiopulmonary standards. He proposes that donors or families should be allowed to choose the definition of death that fits best with their personal values.[12]

Recently, the DDR has been seriously compromised in three protocols involving infants in which the recommended time after the cessation of the heartbeat was reduced from the minimum recommended time of two- to five-minutes to seventy-five seconds.[13] This is an unacceptably dangerous assault on the DDR. The uncertainties of death determination in infants are notoriously formidable. Extrapolations based on these cases are exceedingly perilous and border on the irresponsible.

Also recently, Miller and Truog[14] have expanded their attack on the DDR, calling for its abolition and replacement by the autonomous consent of the donor or his or her surrogate. Their line of reasoning is a utilitarian device: They abolish the DDR, replace it with autonomous choice, and declare that such a move makes removal of vital organs from the donor ethically defensible. Indeed, on their view, this revision is ethically laudable because it removes the "veneer" hiding the fact that both the neurological and cardiopulmonary standards result in killing donors. They reject using the word "killing" as counterproductive, although they admit it could be called killing. Their attempt to justify the taking of vital organs from living donors will undoubtedly be seriously debated.

Relaxation of the DDR is a morally unacceptable and logically specious way to deal with the uncertainties of the criteria for death of the donor. It leaves the choice of the criteria for death to individual preference, amounting to eventual abolition of any stable criteria for death. Some additional dangers are: the use of assisted suicide to facilitate organ donation; legitimizing the use of patients in permanent vegetative states or of "less-than-perfect" infants as donors. It exposes "undeclared" patients to "presumed" consent to donation. Given the expanding cultural and ethical pluralism of the U.S. about all aspects of life and death, eliminating the DDR promises a future of moral and legal chaos. Above all, it exposes the vulnerable or gullible patient to an increased danger of exploitation for the benefit of others.

The need for organs, the desire to prolong life, and the potential "good" to be done are forces difficult to control when death can be defined on one's own—or one's guardian's—terms. As experience has repeatedly shown, personal autonomy without moral constraint ends in divisive moral atomism. As difficult as the search for a common definition of death may be, that difficulty cannot justify abandoning the effort to establish a common definition or manipulating the DDR to meet the need for more organs.

Which Standard Should Be Preferred—the Neurological or the Cardiopulmonary?

Since the 1970s, the dominant criteria for death of the donor have been those of the neurological standard (a heart-beating donor). In recent years, there has been a resurgent interest in the cardiopulmonary standard (a non-heart-beating donor) under the auspices of protocols known as "controlled donation after cardiac death," protocols that have recently received approval of prestigious medical bodies in the United States and Canada.[15] The Council's opinion is that both the neurological and the cardiopulmonary standards are ethically acceptable, but some Council members have expressed reservations about the use of the cardiopulmonary standard in "controlled donation after cardiac death protocols."

In my view, the reasons that favor the neurological standard are not compelling. The clinical tests and signs that support it are as subject to doubt as those of the cardiopulmonary standard. The philosophical arguments for both suffer from the same conceptual and empirical difficulties already identified and examined.

Some favor the neurological standard over the cardiopulmonary standard because of the possibility of auto-resuscitation with the latter. Auto-resuscitation has occurred in rare instances, but not in controlled non-heart-beating protocols if the time after withdrawal of respirator support was five minutes or more.[16]

Others oppose the cardiopulmonary standard because of doubts about possible lack of irreversibility of cardiac function. How, they ask, can a supposedly "dead" heart be transplanted from a "dead" donor and "revived" to function in a recipient?[17] But the fact is that the donated heart is transplanted from a physiological environment that could not support the metabolism of myocardial cells to a physiological environment suitable to cell metabolism. The heart from a patient declared dead by the cardiopulmonary standard can beat when transplanted because autolysis occurs at different rates in different organs. An organ removed when cellular autolysis has not yet advanced to a point that would cause organ failure can function when placed in a physiologically normal, natural or artificial environment that meets its metabolic needs.

Furthermore, if valid, the same argument would apply to other organs as well. Kidneys, intestines, lungs, etc., are taken from donors pronounced "dead" by both the neurological and cardiopulmonary standards. These organs are taken from a supposedly "dead" donor in full expectation that they will function in a recipient.

Taking everything into account, I believe there is as much—or more—moral assurance of death of the donor with the cardiopulmonary as with the neurological standard. In fact, with the cardiopulmonary standard, there is a higher degree of certainty of death than there is with a heart-beating donor, because heart, lung, and brain have all ceased functioning.

Can Transplantation Be Ethically Legitimated?

Do the considerable doubts about both the neurological and cardiopulmonary standards make organ transplantation ethically indefensible? One way to examine this question is as a problem of prudential or practical reason—that is, all things considered, how can we act ethically in the face of relative clinical doubt? This is the context within which many important clinical decisions must be made in modern medicine and have always been made in medicine's past.

Many, if not most, serious clinical decisions must be made in a matrix of concrete, contingent, and uncertain realities in the present and the future. This is why medicine has rightly been called by one of its wisest practitioners "...a science of uncertainty and an art of probability."[18] The moral danger of removing vital organs from a donor whose death is not reasonably certain is significant. However, if absolute certainty is not possible, a sufficient degree of moral certainty to warrant such an action may be attainable if the requirements for prudent decision-making are satisfied.

Prudence in both the ethical and clinical aspects of bedside decisions is an indispensable practical virtue for the good clinician. It is the capability to choose, in any difficult decision, the means that will most closely fit the good intent of the clinical act. Prudence serves the first rule of all ethics, to do good and to avoid evil, even in the most difficult circumstances. Prudence activates two principles of moral action in the face of doubt: the precautionary principle (i.e., when in doubt, act to avoid the gravest danger) and the principle of proportionality (i.e., properly balance the benefits and the burdens of treatment). Prudential reasoning deserves closer attention than it has received in the current debate about the determination of death.

Relative moral certitude does not substitute for scientific certitude. But, properly weighed, it can give a legitimate warrant for necessary action in the face of unavoidable uncertainty. This is the situation within which ordinary decisions in daily life are made. Clinical prudence seeks to avoid both the error of inaction, which would deprive the recipient of a needed transplant, and the error of premature action, which would deprive the donor of life. Fidelity to beneficence and the prudential approach to decisions aim to avoid both the paralysis of inaction and the harmful use of ineffective medical treatments. Prudence must not be confused with self-protective cowardice. It is the decision to act for a good end in the morally optimal way despite persistent uncertainty about the outcome.

Futility in the Decision Process

The moral quality of a non-beating heart donation can be improved as can the degree of compliance with the DDR by use of the principle of futility. When considering the moral quality of a decision to initiate a donation protocol, the relevance of clinical futility deserves attention. Futility is that state in the history of a patient's disease when he or she is beyond medical rescue, i.e., beyond the powers of medical technology to help. Clinical futility is present when any medical intervention is: (1) *ineffective*, i.e., unable to change the natural history of a disease or its trajectory towards death; (2) *non-beneficial*, i.e., unable to satisfy any good or value perceived by the patient or his or her surrogate; and (3) *disproportionately burdensome* to the patient, physically, psychologically, or financially.[19] Balancing the relationship among those three criteria is at the heart of prudent, precautionary, and proportionate action. This formulation accommodates the physician's expertise with respect to effectiveness and the patient's values with respect to benefits, and it results in shared decision-making regarding the proportionality of benefits and burdens.

Care of the patient is *never* futile. Provision of comfort, pain relief, easing of suffering, and palliative care are always morally mandatory. They are the indispensable and absolute requirements for morally valid care at the end of life for every patient. However, under the conditions of ethically legitimate futility, medical interventions may be discontinued. Indeed, if continued, clinically futile medical treatment can convert beneficence into maleficence. Valid use of the principle of futility is *not* medical abandonment. It does include patient participation as well.

When the criteria for clinical futility are properly met and attested to by the attending physician together with the family, the patient's life-support can ethically be removed. Following removal of life-support and cessation of both respiration and cardiac function, initiation of a "controlled donation after cardiac death" (controlled DCD) protocol may begin.

Ethically sensitive controlled DCD recovery protocols are being developed and used by institutions providing transplant services. My purpose is not to compare and contrast those protocols or their comparative ethical acceptability. Some of the ethical constraints by which any transplant protocol may be judged, however, include the following: both the prospective donor and the prospective recipient must be treated as patients in their own right—each with his or her own attending physician whose major concern is the patient's needs and not the needs of the protocol; the donor's physician must, together with the family, determine whether further treatment would be futile; quality of life can be a valid factor only if expressed by the patient or the patient's morally valid surrogate; care and relief of pain and suffering are never futile, nor is palliative care. The usual ethical requirements for morally and legally valid consent must be observed; the declaration of death must be neither premature nor overdue.

The prospective donor and the prospective recipient must therefore be treated in accord with the principle of beneficence. If we grant, as I do, that Jonas's judgment about the imprecision of decisions at the life-death interface is cogent, then his advice to "lean" in the direction of protecting life is ethically sound and grounded in a valid precautionary principle. Within these ethical constraints, the dignity of the donor and recipient, and the benefits of organ transplantation, can be protected. The act of organ donation could retain its moral credibility without compromising care of the donor.

Remaining Ethical Uncertainties

Clinical and ethical uncertainties remain with both brain death and controlled DCD protocols. When the respirator is removed, there is the possibility that electrical activity of the myocardium may return after the prescribed five minute waiting period. Return of electrical activity is not synonymous with effective mechanical pumping. Nevertheless, some may feel constrained to consider cardiopulmonary resuscitation. This possibility can be anticipated by a prior, valid "do not resuscitate" (DNR) order. This order is invoked only when medical treatment is truly futile, death is foreseeable within a short period, and further cardiopulmonary resuscitation can itself be expected to meet the criteria of futility. A valid DNR order implies that death is to be allowed to occur naturally as the final event of an illness whose inevitable natural clinical trajectory is death within a foreseeable interval. Under these circumstances, cardiopulmonary resuscitation would not be in the patient's interest.

The danger of hastening the decision to discontinue treatment is present with both the neurological and the cardiopulmonary standards for determination of death.[*] In both, the only safeguard against such a decision is the ethical fidelity of physicians and families to the patient's welfare. The decision not to resuscitate must be based on the futility of all technical medical procedures, not the need, however great, for a transplantable organ by a particular patient.

Not to be ignored are the social costs of shifting the criteria for organ procurement from brain death to the cardiopulmonary standard. Such a move places the good of the dying potential donor over that of a dying recipient in need of a life-saving organ. This change may result in delays, greater procedural complexity, loss of vitality of the more sensitive organs, and, perhaps, fewer organs

---

[*] One glaring example is a $1.5 million grant over three years to New York City from the federal Health Resources and Services Administration to study the use of a special ambulance fully equipped for removal of organs for transplantation. This vehicle would be rushed to the site of traumatic incidents, ready to remove organs as soon as the donor's death was declared. (Cara Buckley, "City to Explore a Way to Add Organs" (*New York Times* June 1, 2008. Available at http://www.nytimes.com/2008/06/01/nyregion/01organ.html. Accessed December 10, 2008).

available for transplantation. Here, the vexed issue of social versus individual good arises and sharp differences of opinion between and among interested parties seem unavoidable.

I have chosen to give priority to the welfare of the patient before he or she becomes a donor on grounds that harm must not be done even if good comes from it. No person should be sacrificed as a means for the good of another. This is a moral precept that recognizes the intrinsic worth of every human being.

The significant controversies and doubts about when the donor is dead cannot justify abandonment of the DDR. Rather, it should stimulate research into how to extend the viability of potentially transplantable organs. It might also accelerate the process well under way to grow organs extra-corporeally for transplant purposes. This has already been done successfully with at least a diseased urinary bladder and a trachea grown from cells from the patient's body. In the case of the trachea, that organ was removed from a dead donor, stripped of the donor's cells, and a new trachea was formed using the remaining cartilaginous skeleton and the recipient's own stem cells. [20]

Ultimately, the central ethical challenge for any transplantation protocol is to give the gift of life to one human being without taking life away from another. Until the uncertainties and imprecision of the life-death spectrum so clearly recognized by Hans Jonas are dispelled, his moral advice must be our guide for all transplant protocols:

> We do not know with certainty the borderline between life and death, and a definition cannot substitute for knowledge. Moreover, we have sufficient grounds for suspecting that the artificially supported condition of the comatose patient may still be one of life, however reduced—i.e., for doubting that, even with the brain function gone, he is completely dead. In this state of marginal ignorance and doubt the only course to take is to lean over backward toward the side of possible life. [21]

ENDNOTES

[1] Aristotle, *Topics* (155a 18-19) in *The Complete Works of Aristotle, The Revised Oxford Translation, Vol. 1*, ed. Jonathan Barnes (Princeton, New Jersey: Princeton University Press, 1971), 260.

[2] Hans Jonas, "Against the Stream," in *Philosophical Essays, From Ancient Creed to Technological Man*, (Englewood Cliffs, New Jersey: Prentice-Hall, 1974), pp. 132-140. See also *Controversies in the Determination of Death, A White Paper of the President's Council on Bioethics*, 33-37.

[3] Aristotle, *Nicomachean Ethics* (1094b 13-15) in *The Complete Works of Aristotle, The Revised Oxford Translation, Vol. 2*, ed. Jonathan Barnes (Princeton, New Jersey: Princeton University Press, 1971), p.1730

[4] President's Commission for the Study of Ethical Problems in Medicine and Biomedical and Behavioral Research, *Defining Death: Medical, Legal and Ethical Issues in the Determination of Death* (Washington, D.C.: U.S. Government Printing Office, 1981).

[5] *Cf.* D. Alan Shewmon, "The Brain and Somatic Integration: Insights into the Standard Biological Rationale for Equating 'Brain Death' with Death." *Journal of Medicine and Philosophy* 26, no. 5 (2001): 457-78. See also D. Alan Shewmon, "Mental Disconnect: 'Physiological Decapitation" as a Heuristic for Understanding 'Brain Death'," *Working Group on the Signs of Death 11-12 September 2006*, ed. H.E. Msgr. Marcelo Sanchez Sorondo (Vatican City: Pontifica Academia Scientiarum, 2007), pp. 292-333.

[6] *Controversies in the Determination of Death, A White Paper of the President's Council on Bioethics*. See also K. G. Karakatsanis. "'Brain Death': Should It Be Reconsidered?" *Spinal Cord* 46, no. 6 (2008): 396-401.

[7] H. Tristram Engelhardt, Jr., *The Foundations of Bioethics*, 2d ed. (New York: Oxford University Press, 1996), p.242

[8] Plato, *Gorgias* (524b-c), trans. Robin Waterfield (New York: Oxford University Press, 2008), 131.

[9] Plato, *Phaedo* (71d), trans. R. Hackforth (New York: Cambridge University Press, 1972), 64.

[10] See Liang Cheng and David Z. Bostwick, eds., "Decomposition," in *Essentials of Anatomic Pathology 2d ed.* (Totowa, New Jersey: Humana Press, 2005), 87-92; Arpad Vass, "How Long Does Cellular Metabolism Persist After Death?" *Scientific American* September 2008, p. 116; *Cell Death and Differentiation* 15, no. 7 (July 2008).

[11] Robert D. Truog and Franklin G. Miller, "The Dead Donor Rule and Organ Transplantation," *New England Journal of Medicine* 359, no. 7 (August 14, 2008):674-675.

[12] Robert M. Veatch, "Donating Hearts after Cardiac Death – Reversing the Irreversible," *New England Journal of Medicine* 359, no. 7 (August 14, 2008):672-673.

[13] Mark M. Boucek, Christine Mashburn, et al., "Pediatric Heart Transplantation after Declaration of Cardiopulmonary Death," *New England Journal of Medicine* 359, no. 7 (August 14, 2008):709-714. Special Task Force, American Academy of Pediatrics, "Guidelines for the Determination of Brain Death in Children," *Pediatrics* 80 (1987): 298-300.

[14] Franklin G. Miller and Robert D. Truog, "Rethinking the Ethics of Vital Organ Donations," *Hastings center Report* November-December 2008: 38-46.

[15] Institute of Medicine, *Organ Donation: Opportunities for Action* (Washington, D.C.: National Academy Press, 2006; Society of Critical Care Medicine, "Recommendations for Nonheartbeating Organ Donation." *Critical Care Medicine* 29, no. 9 (2001): 1826-31; Joint Commission. "2009 Accreditation Requirements: Accreditation Program: Critical Access Hospital," (2008).

[16] Bruce Ben-David, et al., "Survival after Failed Intra-operative Resuscitation: A Case of the Lazarus Syndrome," *Journal of Anesthesiology and Analgesia* 92 (2001):690-692. See also M.A. Da Vita, "The Death Watch: Certifying Death Using Cardiac Criteria," *Progress in Transplantation* 11, no. 1 (2001):58-66.

[17] Veatch, "Donating Hearts after Cardiac Death."

[18] William Osler, *Sir William Osler Aphorisms; From His Bedside Teachings and Writings, collected by Robert Bennett Bean, edited by William Bennett Bean* (Springfield, Ill.: Charles C. Thomas, Publisher, 1968), p.129.

[19] Edmund D. Pellegrino, "Decisions at the End of Life: The Use and Abuse of the Concept of Futility," in *The Dignity of the Dying Person (Proceedings of the Fifth Assembly of the Pontifical Academy for Life* (February 24-27, 1999), ed. Juan De Dios Vial Correa and Elio Sgreccia (Citta del Vaticano: Libreria Editrice Vaticano, 2000), 219-241. See also Edmund D. Pellegrino, "Futility in Medical Decisions: The Word and the Concept," *Healthcare Ethics Committee Forum* 17, no. 4 (December 2005):308-318.

[20] Paulo Macchiarini, et al., "Clinical Transplantation of a Tissue-Engineered Airway," *The Lancet* on-line November 19, 2008.

[21] Jonas, "Against the Stream," 138.

TOPICAL BIBLIOGRAPHY

TOPICAL BIBLIOGRAPHY

1   Publications of Government Commissions and Professional Societies

1.1   Neurological Standard

Ad Hoc Committee of the Harvard Medical School to Examine the Definition of Brain Death. "A Definition of Irreversible Coma." *JAMA* 205, no. 6 (1968): 337-40.

American Academy of Neurology, Quality Standards Subcommittee. "Practice Parameters for Determining Brain Death in Adults (Summary Statement)." *Neurology* 45, no. 5 (1995): 1012-4.

Institute of Society, Ethics, and the Life Sciences, Task Force on Death and Dying. "Refinements in Criteria for the Determination of Death: An Appraisal." *JAMA* 221, no. 1 (1972): 48-53.

President's Commission for the Study of Ethical Problems in Medicine and Biomedical and Behavioral Research. *Defining Death: Medical, Legal and Ethical Issues in the Determination of Death*. Washington, D.C.: Government Printing Office, 1981.

President's Commission for the Study of Ethical Problems in Medicine and Biomedical and Behavioral Research, Report of the Medical Consultants on the Diagnosis of Death. "Guidelines for the Determination of Death." *JAMA* 246, no. 19 (1981): 2184-6.

Shemie, S. D., C. Doig, B. Dickens, P. Byrne, B. Wheelock, G. Rocker, A. Baker, et al. "Severe Brain Injury to Neurological Determination of Death: Canadian Forum Recommendations." *CMAJ* 174, no. 6 (2006): S1-13.

Task Force for the Determination of Brain Death in Children. "Guidelines for the Determination of Brain Death in Children." *Neurology* 37, no. 6 (1987): 1077-8.

1.2 Donation After Cardiac Death

Bernat, J. L., A. M. D'Alessandro, F. K. Port, T. P. Bleck, S. O. Heard, J. Medina, S. H. Rosenbaum, et al. "Report of a National Conference on Donation after Cardiac Death." *Am J Transplant* 6, no. 2 (2006): 281-91.

Institute of Medicine. *Non-Heart-Beating Organ Transplantation: Medical and Ethical Issues in Procurement.* Washington, D.C.: National Academy Press, 1997.

———. *Non-Heart-Beating Organ Transplantation: Practice and Protocols.* Washington, D.C.: National Academy Press, 2000.

———. *Organ Donation: Opportunities for Action.* Washington, D.C.: National Academy Press, 2006.

Joint Commission. "2009 Accreditation Requirements: Accreditation Program: Critical Access Hospital." 2008.

Shemie, S. D., A. J. Baker, G. Knoll, W. Wall, G. Rocker, D. Howes, J. Davidson, et al. "National Recommendations for Donation after Cardiocirculatory Death in Canada: Donation after Cardiocirculatory Death in Canada." *CMAJ* 175, no. 8 (2006): S1.

Society of Critical Care Medicine. "Recommendations for Non-heartbeating Organ Donation." *Crit Care Med* 29, no. 9 (2001): 1826-31.

2 Critical Literature: The Neurological Standard for Death

2.1 Law, Policy, and History

Bagheri, A. "Organ Transplantation Laws in Asian Countries: A Comparative Study." *Transplant Proc* 37, no. 10 (2005): 4159-62.

Beresford, H. R. "Legal Aspects of Brain Death." In *Brain Death*, edited by E. F. Wijdicks. Philadelphia: Lippincott Williams & Wilkins, 2001.

Capron, A. M., and F. Cate. "Death and Organ Transplantation." In *Treatise on Health Care Law*, edited by R. M. Kaufman, M. G. Macdonald, A. M. Capron, I. M. Birnbaum. New York: Matthew Bender, 1991.

Diringer, M. N., and E. F. Wijdicks. "Brain Death in Historical Perspective." In *Brain Death*, edited by E. F. Wijdicks, 5-27. Philadelphia: Lippincott Williams & Wilkins, 2001.

Lock, M. M. *Twice Dead: Organ Transplants and the Reinvention of Death*. Berkeley: University of California Press, 2002.

Machado, C. "The First Organ Transplant from a Brain-Dead Donor." *Neurology* 64, no. 11 (2005): 1938-42.

Machado, C., J. Kerein, Y. Ferrer, L. Portela, M. de la C. García, and J. M. Manero. "The Concept of Brain Death Did Not Evolve to Benefit Organ Transplants." *J Med Ethics* 33, no. 4 (2007): 197-200.

Pernick, M. S. "Back from the Grave: Recurring Controversies over Defining and Diagnosing Death in History." In *Death: Beyond Whole Brain Criteria*, edited by R. M. Zaner, 17-74. Dordrecht: Kluwer Academic Publishers, 1988.

————. "Brain Death in a Cultural Context: The Reconstruction of Death, 1967-1981." In *The Definition of Death: Contemporary Controversies*, edited by S. J. Youngner, R. M. Arnold, and R. Schapiro, 3-33. Baltimore: The Johns Hopkins University Press, 1999.

Wendler, D., and N. Dickert. "The Consent Process for Cadaveric Organ Procurement: How Does It Work? How Can It Be Improved?" *JAMA* 285, no. 3 (2001): 329-33.

Wijdicks, E. F. "The Neurologist and Harvard Criteria for Brain Death." *Neurology* 61, no. 7 (2003): 970-6.

2.2 Clinical Guidelines, Practice, and Research

Agarwal, R., N. Singh, and D. Gupta. "Is the Patient Brain-Dead?" *Emerg Med J* 23, no. 1 (2006): e5.

Bernat, J. L. "On Irreversibility as a Prerequisite for Brain Death Determination." *Adv Exp Med Biol* 550 (2004): 161-7.

Booth, C. M., R. H. Boone, G. Tomlinson, and A. S. Detsky. "Is This Patient Dead, Vegetative, or Severely Neurologically Impaired? Assessing Outcome for Comatose Survivors of Cardiac Arrest." *JAMA* 291, no. 7 (2004): 870-9.

Ingvar, D. H. "Brain Death—Total Brain Infarction." *Acta Anaesthesiol Scand Suppl* 45 (1971): 129-40.

Karakatsanis K. G. "'Brain Death': Should It Be Reconsidered?" *Spinal Cord* 46, no. 6 (2008): 396-401.

Laureys, S. "Science and Society: Death, Unconsciousness and the Brain." *Nat Rev Neurosci* 6, no. 11 (2005): 899-909.

Laureys, S., A. M. Owen, and N. D. Schiff. "Brain Function in Coma, Vegetative State, and Related Disorders." *Lancet Neurol* 3, no. 9 (2004): 537-46.

Mollaret, P., and M. Goulon. "Le Coma Dépassé." *Rev Neurol (Paris)* 101 (1959): 3-15.

Plum, F. "Clinical Standards and Technological Confirmatory Tests in Diagnosing Brain Death." In *The Definition of Death: Contemporary Controversies*, edited by S. J. Youngner, R. M. Arnold, and R. Schapiro, 34-65. Baltimore: The Johns Hopkins University Press, 1999.

Powner, D. J., and I. M. Bernstein. "Extended Somatic Support for Pregnant Women after Brain Death." *Crit Care Med* 31, no. 4 (2003): 1241-9.

Repertinger, S., W. P. Fitzgibbons, M. F. Omojola, and R. A. Brumback. "Long Survival Following Bacterial Meningitis-Associated Brain Destruction." *J Child Neurol* 21, no. 7 (2006): 591-5.

Silverman, M. E., D. Grove, and C. B. Upshaw, Jr. "Why Does the Heart Beat? The Discovery of the Electrical System of the Heart." *Circulation* 113, no. 23 (2006): 2775-81.

Stedman, T. L. *Stedman's Medical Dictionary*. 26th ed. Baltimore: Lippincott Williams & Wilkins, 1995.

Sundin-Huard, D., and K. Fahy. "The Problems with the Validity of the Diagnosis of Brain Death." *Nurs Crit Care* 9, no. 2 (2004): 64-71.

Waters, C. E., G. French, and M. Burt. "Difficulty in Brainstem Death Testing in the Presence of High Spinal Cord Injury." *Br J Anaesth* 92, no. 5 (2004): 760-4.

Wijdicks, E. F. "The Diagnosis of Brain Death." *N Engl J Med* 344, no. 16 (2001): 1215-21.

———. "Clinical Diagnosis and Confirmatory Testing of Brain Death in Adults." In *Brain Death*, edited by E. F. Wijdicks. Philadelphia: Lippincott Williams & Wilkins, 2001.

Wijdicks, E. F., and J.L. Atkinson. "Pathophysiologic Responses to Brain Death." In *Brain Death*, edited by E. F. Wijdicks. Philadelphia: Lippincott Williams & Wilkins, 2001.

2.2.1 "Donor Management"

Arbour, R. "Clinical Management of the Organ Donor." *AACN Clin Issues* 16, no. 4 (2005): 551-80.

Darby, J. M., K. Stein, A. Grenvik, and S. A. Stuart. "Approach to Management of the Heartbeating 'Brain Dead' Organ Donor." *JAMA* 261, no. 15 (1989): 2222-8.

Dosemeci, L., M. Cengiz, M. Yilmaz, and A. Ramazanoglu. "Frequency of Spinal Reflex Movements in Brain-Dead Patients." *Transplant Proc* 36, no. 1 (2004): 17-9.

Keep, P. J. "Anaesthesia for Organ Donation in the Brainstem Dead." *Anaesthesia* 55, no. 6 (2000): 590.

Saposnik, G., J. A. Bueri, J. Maurino, R. Saizar, and N. S. Garretto. "Spontaneous and Reflex Movements in Brain Death." *Neurology* 54, no. 1 (2000): 221-3.

Wace, J., and M. Kai. "Anaesthesia for Organ Donation in the Brainstem Dead." *Anaesthesia* 55, no. 6 (2000): 590.

Young, P. J., and B. F. Matta. "Anaesthesia for Organ Donation in the Brainstem Dead—Why Bother?" *Anaesthesia* 55, no. 2 (2000): 105-6.

2.2.2 Consistency in Application of Diagnostic Criteria

Powner, D. J., M. Hernandez, and T. E. Rives. "Variability among Hospital Policies for Determining Brain Death in Adults." *Crit Care Med* 32, no. 6 (2004): 1284-8.

Shemie, S. D. "Variability of Brain Death Practices." *Crit Care Med* 32, no. 12 (2004): 2564-5.

Wang, M. Y., P. Wallace, and J. P. Gruen. "Brain Death Documentation: Analysis and Issues." *Neurosurgery* 51, no. 3 (2002): 731-5; discussion 35-6.

Wijdicks, E. F. "Brain Death Worldwide: Accepted Fact but No Global Consensus in Diagnostic Criteria." *Neurology* 58, no. 1 (2002): 20-5.

2.2.3   Pediatrics

Ashwal, S. "Clinical Diagnosis and Confirmatory Testing of Brain Death in Children." In *Brain Death*, edited by E. F. Wijdicks. Philadelphia: Lippincott Williams & Wilkins, 2001.

Banasiak, K. J., and G. Lister. "Brain Death in Children." *Curr Opin Pediatr* 15, no. 3 (2003): 288-93.

Brilli, R. J., and D. Bigos. "Apnea Threshold and Pediatric Brain Death." *Crit Care Med* 28, no. 4 (2000): 1257.

Chang, M. Y., L. A. McBride, and M. A. Ferguson. "Variability in Brain Death Declaration Practices in Pediatric Head Trauma Patients." *Pediatr Neurosurg* 39, no. 1 (2003): 7-9.

Mejia, R. E., and M. M. Pollack. "Variability in Brain Death Determination Practices in Children." *JAMA* 274, no. 7 (1995): 550-3.

Shemie, S. D., M. M. Pollack, M. Morioka, and S. Bonner. "Diagnosis of Brain Death in Children." *Lancet Neurol* 6, no. 1 (2007): 87-92.

Vardis, R., and M. M. Pollack. "Increased Apnea Threshold in a Pediatric Patient with Suspected Brain Death." *Crit Care Med* 26, no. 11 (1998): 1917-9.

2.2.4 Withholding or Withdrawing Life Support and Persistent Vegetative State

Keenan, S. P., K. D. Busche, L. M. Chen, L. McCarthy, K. J. Inman, and W. J. Sibbald. "A Retrospective Review of a Large Cohort of Patients Undergoing the Process of Withholding or Withdrawal of Life Support." *Crit Care Med* 25, no. 8 (1997): 1324-31.

Owen, A. M., M. R. Coleman, M. Boly, M. H. Davis, S. Laureys, and J. D. Pickard. "Detecting Awareness in the Vegetative State." *Science* 313, no. 5792 (2006): 1402.

————. "Using Functional Magnetic Resonance Imaging to Detect Covert Awareness in the Vegetative State." *Arch Neurol* 64, no. 8 (2007): 1098-1102.

Pellegrino, E. D. "Decisions to Withdraw Life-Sustaining Treatment: A Moral Algorithm," *JAMA*, 283, no. 8 (2000): 1065-7.

————. "Futility in Medical Decisions: The Word and the Concept." *HEC Forum* 17, no. 4 (2005): 308-18.

Prendergast, T. J., and J. M. Luce. "Increasing Incidence of Withholding and Withdrawal of Life Support from the Critically Ill." *Am J Respir Crit Care Med* 155, no. 1 (1997): 15-20.

Smedira, N. G., B. H. Evans, L. S. Grais, N. H. Cohen, B. Lo, M. Cooke, W. P. Schecter, et al. "Withholding and Withdrawal of Life Support from the Critically Ill." *N Engl J Med* 322, no. 5 (1990): 309-15.

2.3 Ethical Debate

Bagheri, A. "Individual Choice in the Definition of Death." *J Med Ethics* 33, no. 3 (2007): 146-9.

————. "Criticism of 'Brain Death' Policy in Japan." *Kennedy Inst Ethics J* 13, no. 4 (2003): 359-72.

Bartlett, E. T, and S. J. Younger. "Human Death and the Destruction of the Neocortex." In *Death: Beyond Whole Brain Criteria*, edited by R. M. Zaner. Dordrecht: Kluwer Academic Publishers, 1988.

Bernat, J. L. "The Whole-Brain Concept of Death Remains Optimum Public Policy." *J Law Med Ethics* 34, no. 1 (2006): 35-43.

————. "The Biophilosophical Basis of Whole-Brain Death." *Soc Philos Policy* 19, no. 2 (2002): 324-42.

————. "Refinements in the Definition and Criterion of Death." In *The Definition of Death: Contemporary Controversies*, edited by S. J. Youngner, R. M. Arnold, and R. Schapiro, 83-92. Baltimore: The Johns Hopkins University Press, 1999.

Bernat, J. L., C. M. Culver, and B. Gert. "On the Definition and Criterion of Death." *Ann Intern Med* 94, no. 3 (1981): 389-94.

Browne, A. "Whole-Brain Death Reconsidered." *J Med Ethics* 9, no. 1 (1983): 28-31, 44.

Byrne, P. A., S. O'Reilly, and P. M. Quay. "Brain Death—an Opposing Viewpoint." *JAMA* 242, no. 18 (1979): 1985-90.

Byrne, P. A., S. O'Reilly, P. M. Quay, and P.W. Salsich. "Brain Death—the Patient, the Physician, and Society." In *Beyond Brain Death: The Case against Brain Based Criteria for Human Death*, edited by M. Potts, P. A. Byrne, and R. G. Nigles. Dordrecht: Kluwer Academic Publishers, 2000.

Capron, A. M. "Brain Death—Well Settled Yet Still Unresolved." *N Engl J Med* 344, no. 16 (2001): 1244-6.

———. "The Bifurcated Legal Standard for Determining Death: Does It Work?" In *The Definition of Death: Contemporary Controversies*, edited by S. J. Youngner, R. M. Arnold, and R. Schapiro, 117-36. Baltimore: The Johns Hopkins University Press, 1999.

———. "The Report of the President's Commission on the Uniform Determination of Death Act." In *Death: Beyond Whole Brain Criteria*, edited by R. M. Zaner. Dordrecht: Kluwer Academic Publishers, 1988.

———. "The Purpose of Death: A Reply to Professor Dworkin." *Indiana Law J* 48, no. 4 (1973): 640-6.

Capron, A. M., and L. R. Kass. "Statutory Definition of Standards for Determining Human Death—Appraisal and a Proposal." *University of Pennsylvania Law Review* 121, no. 1 (1972): 87-118.

Charo, R. A. "Dusk, Dawn and Defining Death: Legal Classifications and Biological Categories." In *The Definition of Death: Contemporary Controversies*, edited by S. J. Youngner, R. M. Arnold, and R. Schapiro, 277-92. Baltimore: The Johns Hopkins University Press, 1999.

Chiong, W. "Brain Death Without Definitions." *Hastings Cent Rep* 35, no. 6 (2005): 20-30.

Cranford, R. "Even the Dead Are Not Terminally Ill Anymore." *Neurology* 51, no. 6 (1998): 1530-1.

Dagi, F. T., and R. Kaufman. "Clarifying the Discussion on Brain Death." *J Med Philos* 26, no. 5 (2001): 503-25.

Doig, C. J., and E. Burgess. "Brain Death: Resolving Inconsistencies in the Ethical Declaration of Death." *Can J Anaesth* 50, no. 7 (2003): 725-31.

DuBois, J. M. "Organ Transplantation: An Ethical Road Map." *Natl Cathol Bioeth Q* 2, no. 3 (2002): 413-53.

DuBois, J. M., and E. E. Anderson. "Attitudes Toward Death Criteria and Organ Donation among Healthcare Personnel and the General Public." *Prog Transplant* 16, no. 1 (2006): 65-73.

Dworkin, R. B. "Death in Context." *Indiana Law J* 48, no. 4 (1973): 623-39.

Eberl, J. T. "A Thomistic Understanding of Human Death." *Bioethics* 19, no. 1 (2005): 29-48.

Emanuel, L. L. "Reexamining Death. The Asymptotic Model and a Bounded Zone Definition." *Hastings Cent Rep* 25, no. 4 (1995): 27-35.

Furton, E. J. "Brain Death, the Soul, and Organic Life." *Natl Cathol Bioeth Q* 2, no. 3 (2002): 455-70.

Gaylin, W. "Harvesting the Dead." *Harpers* 249, no. 1492 (1974): 23-28.

Gervais, K. G. *Redefining Death.* New Haven: Yale University Press, 1986.

Haddow, G. "The Phenomenology of Death, Embodiment and Organ Transplantation." *Sociol Health Illn* 27, no. 1 (2005): 92-113.

Halevy, A., and B. Brody. "Brain Death: Reconciling Definitions, Criteria, and Tests." *Ann Intern Med* 119, no. 6 (1993): 519-25.

Jonas, H. "Against the Stream." In *Philosophical Essays: From Ancient Creed to Technological Man.* Englewood Cliffs, NJ: Prentice-Hall, 1974.

Kass, L. R. "Death as an Event: A Commentary on Robert Morison." *Science* 173, no. 998 (1971): 698-702.

Korein, J. "The Problem of Brain Death: Development and History." *Ann NY Acad Sci* 315 (1978): 19-38.

Korein, J., and C. Machado. "Brain Death: Updating a Valid Concept for 2004." *Adv Exp Med Biol* 550 (2004): 1-14.

Lizza, J. P. "The Conceptual Basis for Brain Death Revisited: Loss of Organic Integration or Loss of Consciousness?" *Adv Exp Med Biol* 550 (2004): 51-9.

————. *Persons, Humanity, and the Definition of Death*. Baltimore, Md.: Johns Hopkins University Press, 2006.

May, W. "Attitudes Toward the Newly Dead." *Stud Hastings Cent* 1, no. 1 (1973): 3-13.

Meilaender, G. "Terra Es Animata: On Having a Life." *Hastings Cent Rep* 23, no. 4 (1993): 25-32.

Morioka, M. "Reconsidering Brain Death: A Lesson from Japan's Fifteen Years of Experience." *Hastings Cent Rep* 31, no. 4 (2001): 41-6.

Morison, R. S. "Death: Process or Event?" *Science* 173, no. 998 (1971): 694-8.

Nigles, R. G. "Organ Transplantation, Brain Death, and the Slippery Slope: A Neurosurgeon's Perspective." In *Beyond Brain Death: The Case against Brain Based Criteria for Human Death*, edited by M. Potts, P. A. Byrne, and R. G. Nigles. Dordrecht: Kluwer Academic Publishers, 2000.

Pallis, C. "On the Brainstem Criterion of Death." In *The Definition of Death: Contemporary Controversies*, edited by S. J. Youngner, R. M. Arnold, and R. Schapiro, 93-100. Baltimore: The Johns Hopkins University Press, 1999.

————. "Further Thoughts on Brainstem Death." *Anaesth Intensive Care* 23, no. 1 (1995): 20-3.

Pallis, C., and D. H. Harley. *ABC of Brainstem Death*. Second ed. London: BMJ Publishing Group, 1996.

Potts, M. "A Requiem for Whole Brain Death: A Response to D. Alan Shewmon's 'The Brain and Somatic Integration'." *J Med Philos* 26, no. 5 (2001): 479-91.

Ramsey, P. *The Patient as Person*. Second ed. New Haven: Yale University Press, 2002.

Rosen, N. "A Fresh Perspective on PVS and Brain Death." Paper presented at the Annual meeting of the American Society for Bioethics and Humanities, Washington, DC, 2007.

Seifert, J. "Brain Death and Euthanasia." In *Beyond Brain Death: The Case against Brain Based Criteria for Human Death*, edited by M. Potts, P. A. Byrne, and R. G. Nigles. Dordrecht: Kluwer Academic Publishers, 2000.

Shewmon, D. A. "The Brain and Somatic Integration: Insights into the Standard Biological Rationale for Equating 'Brain Death' with Death." *J Med Philos* 26, no. 5 (2001): 457-78.

————. "Spinal Shock and 'Brain Death': Somatic Pathophysiological Equivalence and Implications for the Integrative-Unity Rationale." *Spinal Cord* 37, no. 5 (1999): 313-24.

————. "Chronic 'Brain Death': Meta-Analysis and Conceptual Consequences." *Neurology* 51, no. 6 (1998): 1538-45.

————. "Recovery from 'Brain Death': A Neurologist's Apologia." *Linacre Q* 64, no. 1 (1997): 30-96.

Siminoff, L. A., C. Burant, and S. J. Youngner. "Death and Organ Procurement: Public Beliefs and Attitudes." *Kennedy Inst Ethics J* 14, no. 3 (2004): 217-34.

Smith, D. R. "Legal Issues Leading to the Notion of Neocortical Death." In *Death: Beyond Whole Brain Criteria*, edited by R. M. Zaner. Dordrecht: Kluwer Academic Publishers, 1988.

Spike, J. "Brain Death, Pregnancy, and Posthumous Motherhood." *J Clin Ethics* 10, no. 1 (1999): 57-65.

Spike, J., and J. Greenlaw. "Ethics Consultation: Persistent Brain Death and Religion: Must a Person Believe in Death to Die?" *J Law Med Ethics* 23, no. 3 (1995): 291-4.

Veatch, R. M. "The Death of Whole-Brain Death: The Plague of the Disaggregators, Somaticists, and Mentalists." *J Med Philos* 30, no. 4 (2005): 353-78.

———. "The Conscience Clause: How Much Individual Choice in Defining Death Can Our Society Tolerate?" In *The Definition of Death: Contemporary Controversies*, edited by S. J. Youngner, R. M. Arnold, and R. Schapiro, 137-60. Baltimore: The Johns Hopkins University Press, 1999.

———. "The Impending Collapse of the Whole-Brain Definition of Death." *Hastings Cent Rep* 23, no. 4 (1993): 18-24.

———. "Brain Death and Slippery Slopes." *J Clin Ethics* 3, no. 3 (1992): 181-7.

White, P. D. "Should the Law Define Death?—A Genuine Question." In *Death: Beyond Whole Brain Criteria*, edited by R. M. Zaner, 101-09. Dordrecht: Kluwer Academic Publishers, 1988.

Wijdicks, E. F., and J. L. Bernat. "Chronic 'Brain Death': Meta-Analysis and Conceptual Consequences." *Neurology* 53, no. 6 (1999): 1369-70; Author Reply 71-2.

Wikler, D., and A. J. Weisbard. "Appropriate Confusion over 'Brain Death'." *JAMA* 261, no. 15 (1989): 2246.

Youngner, S. J., C. S. Landefeld, C. J. Coulton, B. W. Juknialis, and M. Leary. "'Brain Death' and Organ Retrieval. A Cross-Sectional Survey of Knowledge and Concepts among Health Professionals." *JAMA* 261, no. 15 (1989): 2205-10.

Zamperetti, N., R. Bellomo, C. A. Defanti, and N. Latronico. "Irreversible Apnoeic Coma 35 Years Later. Towards a More Rigorous Definition of Brain Death?" *Intensive Care Med* 30, no. 9 (2004): 1715-22.

Zaner, R. M. "Brains and Persons: A Critique of Veatch's View." In *Death: Beyond Whole Brain Criteria*, edited by R. M. Zaner, 187-97. Dordrecht: Kluwer Academic Publishers, 1988.

3   Critical Literature: Donation After Cardiac Death

3.1   Law, Policy, and History

DeVita, M. A., and J. V. Snyder. "Development of the University of Pittsburgh Medical Center Policy for the Care of Terminally Ill Patients Who May Become Organ Donors after Death Following the Removal of Life Support." *Kennedy Inst Ethics J* 3, no. 2 (1993): 131-43.

DeVita, M. A., J. V. Snyder, and A. Grenvik. "History of Organ Donation by Patients with Cardiac Death." *Kennedy Inst Ethics J* 3, no. 2 (1993): 113-29.

Zawistowski, C. A., and M. A. DeVita. "Non-Heartbeating Organ Donation: A Review." *J Intensive Care Med* 18, no. 4 (2003): 189-97.

3.2   Clinical Guidelines, Practice, and Research

Abt, P. L., N. M. Desai, M. D. Crawford, L. M. Forman, J. W. Markmann, K. M. Olthoff, and J. F. Markmann. "Survival Following Liver Transplantation from Non-Heart-Beating Donors." *Ann Surg* 239, no. 1 (2004): 87-92.

Boucek, M. M., C. Mashburn, S. M. Dunn, R. Frizell, L. Edwards, B. Pietra, and D. Campbell. "Pediatric Heart Transplantation after Declaration of Cardiocirculatory Death." *N Engl J Med* 359, no. 7 (2008): 709-14.

Cooper, J. T., L. T. Chin, N. R. Krieger, L. A. Fernandez, D. P. Foley, Y. T. Becker, J. S. Odorico, S. J. Knechtle, M. Kalayoglu, H. W. Sollinger, and A. M. D'Alessandro. "Donation after Cardiac Death: The University of Wisconsin Experience with Renal Transplantation." *Am J Transplant* 4, no. 9 (2004): 1490-4.

D'Alessandro, A. M., L. A. Fernandez, L. T. Chin, B. D. Shames, N. A. Turgeon, D. L. Scott, A. Di Carlo, et al. "Donation after Cardiac Death: The University of Wisconsin Experience." *Ann Transplant* 9, no. 1 (2004): 68-71.

Doshi, M. D., and L. G. Hunsicker. "Short- and Long-Term Outcomes with the Use of Kidneys and Livers Donated after Cardiac Death." *Am J Transplant* 7, no. 1 (2007): 122-9.

Foley, D. P., L. A. Fernandez, G. Leverson, L. T. Chin, N. Krieger, J. T. Cooper, B. D. Shames, et al. "Donation after Cardiac Death: The University of Wisconsin Experience with Liver Transplantation." *Ann Surg* 242, no. 5 (2005): 724-31.

Kelso, C. M., L. J. Lyckholm, P. J. Coyne, and T. J. Smith. "Palliative Care Consultation in the Process of Organ Donation after Cardiac Death." *J Palliat Med* 10, no. 1 (2007): 118-26.

Lewis, J., J. Peltier, H. Nelson, W. Snyder, K. Schneider, D. Steinberger, M. Anderson, et al. "Development of the University of Wisconsin Donation after Cardiac Death Evaluation Tool." *Prog Transplant* 13, no. 4 (2003): 265-73.

3.3   Ethical Debate

Aulisio, M. P., M. Devita, and D. Luebke. "Taking Values Seriously: Ethical Challenges in Organ Donation and Transplantation for Critical Care Professionals." *Crit Care Med* 35, no. 2 Suppl (2007): S95-101.

Bernat, J. L. "The Boundaries of Organ Donation after Circulatory Death." *N Engl J Med* 359, no. 7 (2008): 669-71.

———. "Are Organ Donors after Cardiac Death Really Dead?" *J Clin Ethics* 17, no. 2 (2006): 122-32.

Campbell, M. L., and L. J. Weber. "Procuring Organs from a Non-Heart-Beating Cadaver: Commentary on a Case Report." *Kennedy Inst Ethics J* 5, no. 1 (1995): 35-42; discussion 43-9.

Caplan, A. L. "The Telltale Heart: Public Policy and the Utilization of Non-Heart-Beating Donors." *Kennedy Inst Ethics J* 3, no. 2 (1993): 251-62.

DeVita, M. A., J. V. Snyder, R. M. Arnold, and L. A. Siminoff. "Observations of Withdrawal of Life-Sustaining Treatment from Patients Who Became Non-Heart-Beating Organ Donors." *Crit Care Med* 28, no. 6 (2000): 1709-12.

DeVita, M. A., R. Vukmir, J. V. Snyder, and C. Graziano. "Non-Heart-Beating Organ Donation: A Reply to Campbell and Weber." *Kennedy Inst Ethics J* 5, no. 1 (1995): 43-9.

Doig, C. J., and G. Rocker. "Retrieving Organs from Non-Heart-Beating Organ Donors: A Review of Medical and Ethical Issues." *Can J Anaesth* 50, no. 10 (2003): 1069-76.

DuBois, J. M. "Is Organ Procurement Causing the Death of Patients?" *Issues Law Med* 18, no. 1 (2002): 21-41.

———. "Intention, Action, and the Dead Donor Rule: Commentary on Spike." *J Clin Ethics* 11, no. 1 (2000): 78-84; discussion 92-3.

Lynn, J. "Are the Patients Who Become Organ Donors Under the Pittsburgh Protocol for 'Non-Heart-Beating Donors' Really Dead?" *Kennedy Inst Ethics J* 3, no. 2 (1993): 167-78.

Lynn, J., and R. Cranford. "The Persisting Perplexities in the Determination of Death." In *The Definition of Death: Contemporary Controversies*, edited by S. J. Youngner, R. M. Arnold, and R. Schapiro, 101-14. Baltimore: The Johns Hopkins University Press, 1999.

Mandell, M. S., S. Zamudio, D. Seem, L. J. McGaw, G. Wood, P. Liehr, A. Ethier, and A. M. D'Alessandro. "National Evaluation of Healthcare Provider Attitudes Toward Organ Donation after Cardiac Death." *Crit Care Med* 34, no. 12 (2006): 2952-8.

Robertson, J. A. "Policy Issues in a Non-Heart-Beating Donor Protocol." *Kennedy Inst Ethics J* 3, no. 2 (1993): 241-50.

Solomon, M. Z. "Donation after Cardiac Death: Non-Heart-Beating Organ Donation Deserves a Green Light and Hospital Oversight." *Anesthesiology* 98, no. 3 (2003): 601-2.

Spike, J. "Controlled NHBD Protocol for a Fully Conscious Person: When Death Is Intended as an End in Itself and It Has Its Own End." *J Clin Ethics* 11, no. 1 (2000): 73-7.

Veatch, R. M. "Donating Hearts after Cardiac Death—Reversing the Irreversible." *N Engl J Med* 359, no. 7 (2008): 672-3.

Van Norman, G. A. "Another Matter of Life and Death: What Every Anesthesiologist Should Know About the Ethical, Legal, and Policy Implications of the Non-Heart-Beating Cadaver Organ Donor." *Anesthesiology* 98, no. 3 (2003): 763-73.

Youngner, S. J., R. M. Arnold, and M. A. DeVita. "When Is 'Dead'?" *Hastings Cent Rep* 29, no. 6 (1999): 14-21.

Zamperetti, N., R. Bellomo, and C. Ronco. "Defining Death in Non-Heart Beating Organ Donors." *J Med Ethics* 29, no. 3 (2003): 182-5.

4   Critical Literature: The Dead Donor Rule

Arnold, R. M., and S. J. Youngner. "The Dead Donor Rule: Should We Stretch It, Bend It, or Abandon It?" *Kennedy Inst Ethics J* 3, no. 2 (1993): 263-78.

Campbell, C. S. "Harvesting the Living? Separating 'Brain Death' and Organ Transplantation." *Kennedy Inst Ethics J* 14, no. 3 (2004): 301-18.

Crowley-Matoka, M., and R. M. Arnold. "The Dead Donor Rule: How Much Does the Public Care...And How Much Should We Care?" *Kennedy Inst Ethics J* 14, no. 3 (2004): 319-32.

Fost, N. "Reconsidering the Dead Donor Rule: Is It Important That Organ Donors Be Dead?" *Kennedy Inst Ethics J* 14, no. 3 (2004): 249-60.

———. "The Unimportance of Death." In *The Definition of Death: Contemporary Controversies*, edited by S. J. Youngner, R. M. Arnold, and R. Schapiro, 161-78. Baltimore: The Johns Hopkins University Press, 1999.

Kerridge, I. H., P. Saul, M. Lowe, J. McPhee, and D. Williams. "Death, Dying and Donation: Organ Transplantation and the Diagnosis of Death." *J Med Ethics* 28, no. 2 (2002): 89-94.

Menikoff, J. "The Importance of Being Dead: Non-Heart-Beating Organ Donation." *Issues Law Med* 18, no. 1 (2002): 3-20.

Truog, R. D. "Brain Death—Too Flawed to Endure, Too Ingrained to Abandon." *J Law Med Ethics* 35, no. 2 (2007): 273-81.

————. "Is It Time to Abandon Brain Death?" *Hastings Cent Rep* 27, no. 1 (1997): 29-37.

Truog, R. D., and F. G. Miller. "The Dead Donor Rule and Organ Transplantation." *N Engl J Med* 359, no. 7 (2008): 674-5.

Truog, R. D., and W. M. Robinson. "Role of Brain Death and the Dead-Donor Rule in the Ethics of Organ Transplantation." *Crit Care Med* 31, no. 9 (2003): 2391-6.

Youngner, S. J., and R. M. Arnold. "Philosophical Debates About the Definition of Death: Who Cares?" *J Med Philos* 26, no. 5 (2001): 527-37.

❦